Eat to Beat Disease

Eat to Beat Disease

FOODS MEDICINAL QUALITIES

Catherine J Frompovich

Copyright ©2016 Catherine J Frompovich
All rights reserved.

ISBN: 1532840705
ISBN: 9781532840708
Library of Congress Control Number: 2016906818
CreateSpace Independent Publishing Platform
North Charleston, South Carolina

Cover Art: Cartoon of *A Man Choosing Between Healthy And Fast Foods* ©Kraphix / Dreamstime.com

The information in this book is not meant to be diagnostic, prescriptive, or defamatory. Nor is the information or the book intended to replace medical advice. The book is offered for information-sharing purposes and relates some of the author's experiences as a retired practicing *natural* nutritionist, researcher, journalist, plus her personal opinions and comments. All information is presented for education sharing purposes and in keeping with the U.S. Copyright Fair Use provisions. The contents of this book should not be used as, nor to give, medical advice. The purpose of the book is to acquaint readers with food information and research, and to encourage readers to investigate the primary role that food contributes to maintaining optimum health. If readers choose to consider any information in this book, the author and publisher assume no responsibility for readers' choices or courses of action taken.

Comments About
Eat to Beat Disease, Food's Medicinal Qualities

"An apple a day keeps the doctor away." You've heard this saying your whole life. It's stuck around so long because it's true.

It can also be said that whole foods (fruits and vegetables, especially eaten raw) every day will keep the doctor away. If more Americans adopted a diet that was actually healthy – one of mostly fruits and vegetables, just like mom suggested while growing up – and avoid processed foods designed to tempt them, including meats loaded with hormones and antibiotics, there would be much less disease and obesity.

Unfortunately, mainstream "health" advice leads most people down the primrose path toward fake foods with no trace of nutrients in them. These processed, already prepared foods we are coerced into buying are incomplete foods, mostly dead and unable to support life.

In addition to promoting obesity, eating a diet predominated by meats and processed foods leads to acidity in the body, disease, and death.

Obesity and acidity, and their associated diseases like high cholesterol, high blood pressure, cancer, and diabetes, could be virtually wiped away if everyone ate properly.

That's why this book is so important.

Bob Livingston, Editor
The Bob Livingston Letter™
Personal Liberty Digest™

In the age we live in, where 9th grade math was at one time college algebra thirty years ago, so has the food we eat changed that much. In as much change that has occurred, our medical profession has no clue as to what technology has done to the food chain as it currently is being presented. As a rule in my 35 years of practice, the average medical professional is clueless to the vast amount of common sense contained in this book.

As this common sense approach seems logical to those that are the holistic (anti-GMO) movement, there is no teaching of nutrition of any quality in the current school systems being run on tight budgets where reading, writing, and math are the core teaching and nutrition, home economics, and cooking classes are a thing of the past.

As life styles have changed and families are now comprised of two working household members, the kitchen now is just a place where the microwave produces things that taste good, without nutrition, and this is now the norm.

The concepts in this book should be taught starting at the 4th grade level, and no child should be allowed to get out of elementary school without a passing grade on this level of food education.

Catherine does a great job of summarizing where we have ended up with technology and no common sense about what the human body needs as opposed to how much profits can be made by another man on the sickness of others. Catherine has done a great job at summarizing what is needed by everyone to be healthier.

Dr. Richard N. Olree Jr.

This is a great book! Catherine is a REAL and WHOLE FOODs aficionado. Her wealth of food knowledge, and its bodily impact, is nothing short of breathtaking! As a thorough researcher, and experienced clinician, who has helped thousands recover their health, she's a premier go-to person for what's important in food choice and also, just as importantly, how we benefit by making those choices. Catherine rightfully promotes *REAL FOOD foods—not synthetic chemical analogs*—as the true foundation of health and the fuel of life.

Eat to Beat Disease, whether read cover-to-cover or used as a reference for specific information, is absolutely unequaled in the marketplace. Broad application of its knowledge would make history of most disease. Catherine has given us superb tools for total health transformation—we only have to apply them.

Laraine C. Abbey-Katzev, RN Emeritus
MS Biology/Clinical Nutrition
Certified Nutrition Specialist

For the discerning reader, Catherine Frompovich's literary offering in this book is a treasure-trove of statistical health related data and nutritional information. Her ability to describe intricate biochemical functions in plain language that anyone can apply to their dietary schedule to improve health and bodily functions is one of the main educational advantages offered here. Almost all diseases are directly related to what we eat or do not eat. Disease has a cause, and this book is dedicated to solving the cause of disease and not just to treat the symptoms.

Robert E. Jenkins, D.C., M.S., DACBN

Some time ago, I took advantage of a literary license earned by having hosted over a thousand editions of the syndicated *Food Chain Radio Show* to pronounce my very own "Three Laws of the Food Chain," the third law being *Cheap Food Isn't!* In fact, they make food cheap by taking the nutrients out of it and by subsidizing its true cost of production, thus the cheap food they promise is really the expensive food they deliver. Catherine Frompovich takes up arms against the cheap food of industrial agriculture with *Eat to Beat Disease.* Read it. Arm yourself. Survive and thrive!

Michael Olson / Host, Food Chain Radio / Author, MetroFarm

This new book by the prolific author, Catherine Frompovich, is a densely packed, but highly readable, account of how to stay healthy by eating well. In addition to telling us why processed foods are bad, she also addresses the important, but often neglected, issue that genetically modified foods promote toxic herbicides. There's lots of good advice also about healthy herbs, probiotics, vitamin-rich foods, etc. Many great recipes scattered throughout.

Stephanie Seneff, PhD, MIT Senior Research Scientist

Eat to Beat Disease: Foods Medicinal Qualities is the food conversation you won't want to miss! The Internet can create confusion about making food work for you - but Frompovich breaks it all down in such a fun way that it feels like pleasure-reading as much as detailed research.

Heather Callaghan, Editor-in-Chief, NaturalBlaze.com

This concise, easy to use book should be taught in every school and used as a reference in every kitchen, if we are to avoid the increasingly high cost of healthcare in this country.

Richard P Milner, Executive Director, Public Affairs Media, Inc.

Words of Wisdom about Food

The first wealth is health.
Ralph Waldo Emerson

If you can't pronounce it, don't eat it.
Common sense

An apple a day keeps the doctor away.
Proverb

Let food be thy medicine and medicine be thy food.
Hippocrates

Our bodies are our gardens – our wills are our gardeners.
William Shakespeare

From the bitterness of disease man learns the sweetness of health.
Catalan Proverb

He who takes medicine and neglects to diet wastes the skill of his doctors.
Chinese Proverb

The food you eat can be either the safest and most powerful form of medicine or the slowest form of poison.
Ann Wigmore

Any food that requires enhancing by the use of chemical substances should in no way be considered a food.
John H. Tobe

The doctor of the future will no longer treat the human frame with drugs, but rather will cure and prevent disease with nutrition.
Thomas Edison

You can't poison a body into wellness.
Catherine J Frompovich

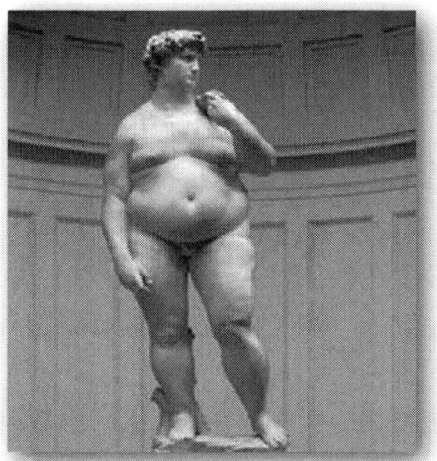

David after 2 years on tour in the USA

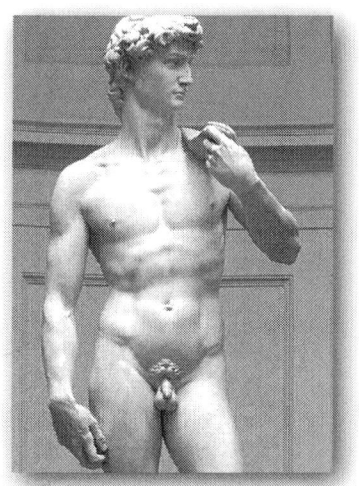

Michelangelo's DAVID
Michelangelo Buonarroti
Carved Between 1501- 1504 AD from one single block of Carrara marble
Accademia Gallery, Florence, Italy

In 2009, *The B.S. Report* posted the above joke photograph of Michelangelo's "David" statue characterizing how David porked up after spending two years on tour in the United States of America.

It's an obvious parody depicting the SAD (sick American diet) food choices and nutritional status in the USA.[1]

The author wishes she knew whom to congratulate for possessing such great computer skills plus insights into the harms of factory-produced, chemicalized, processed, and fast foods.

---

1 https://thebsreport.wordpress.com/2009/09/23/joke-pic-of-the-night-michelangelos-statue-david-being-returned-to-italy/

A Word of Thanks

It is with great admiration that I acknowledge, and thank, everyone who's contributed to the brilliant, but relatively late-blooming, science of nutrition and how food works in the human organism. Thank you to all researchers and authors whose works I have cited, as your efforts have contributed to the ever-growing library and science about something everyone takes for granted, the food we put into our mouths.

I believe in sharing information, the seeds of knowledge are planted.

Who knows what those seeds will produce. I only can hope that they will spring up to help eaters realize that you inadvertently, and metaphorically speaking, may be digging your grave with your very own dinner fork.

Catherine J Frompovich

Table of Contents

Comments About
Eat to Beat Disease, Foods Medicinal Qualities · · · · · · · · · · · · · · · · · v
Words of Wisdom about Food · xi
A Word of Thanks · xv
Foreword · xix
Preface · xxiii
Introduction · xxvii

What's the Premise Behind "There's a science to eating?" · · · · · · · · · · 1
What's the Cause of Most Diseases? · 13
What's Trending Health-wise with Baby-boomers? · · · · · · · · · · · · · 15
What Goes In Must Come Out: A necessary discussion about poop · · 21
Probiotics and Prebiotics: Do you know the difference? · · · · · · · · · 33
Sugar: Is it as sweet a treat as you think? · 37
Do You Have a Sugar Addiction? · 47
The Effects of Food Processing on Nutrients · · · · · · · · · · · · · · · · · 51
Can Food Reduce or Eliminate Pain? · 54
Which Foods Help the Body Most in Managing Certain Diseases? · · · 65
Miscellaneous Diseases Affected by Diet and Nutrition · · · · · · · · · · 70
What's the Story about Toxic Sprays Used on Crops? · · · · · · · · · · · 78
Is There Such a Disorder as "Toxic Body Syndrome"? · · · · · · · · · · · 82
What Role Does Diet Play Regarding Cancer? · · · · · · · · · · · · · · · · 90

HPV Vaccine Reactions: What can someone expect from
diet and nutrition? · 94
Enzymes, Powerful 'Sparkplugs' in Food · 100
The Incredible, Edible B-complex Vitamins: The nutritional
enzyme system enablers for cell metabolism · · · · · · · · · · · · · · · · 107
The Energy Vitamins Everyone Overlooks · · · · · · · · · · · · · · · · · · · 109
Fermented Foods: What do they have to do with
maintaining good health? · 118
Protein, the Building Blocks of Life · 122
GMOs: Genetically modified organisms called 'phood' · · · · · · · · 131
Food Buying, Storing, and Preparation · 143
A Greasy Story about Cooking Oils · 156
EFAs: The fats you really need—Essential Fatty Acids · · · · · · · · 164
Food Families and Allergies · 171
Foods High in Antioxidants · 178
Beans: That wonderful "musical" fruit · 181
Grains: What's to eat besides wheat? · 198
Ice Cream That Can Be Nutritious · 206
The Mineral Iron · 210
M-E-A-T: Do you really want to know what happens to it? · · · · · 212
Medicinal Mushrooms: Fact or fiction? · 219
Smoothies: A fresh start to your day · 229
Soup, the Ultimate Comfort Food · 235
Healthful Snacks – When You Are Ready for Them · · · · · · · · · · · 249
Quick Tips for Healthful Eating · 253
How to Expand Your Knowledge about Nutrition,
Health, and Healing · 256
Filing Consumer Complaints about Food Products · · · · · · · · · · · 259
Recipes from Catherine's Kitchen · 260

Catherine's After Thoughts · 282
About the Author · 287

Foreword

The commonly held belief that modern diseases, like cancer, just spontaneously appear without cause is rooted in unscientific, irrational thinking. Yet, it's exactly what most patients are told when they are diagnosed with cancer. "There's nothing you could have done to prevent it," they're often told by their ill-informed oncologists, who are functionally little more than chemotherapy drug dispensaries pretending to be doctors.

This idea that disease appears without cause is little more than medical voodoo... or perhaps it's better stated as "scientific mysticism." It discards any link between foods and health outcomes, casting aside the simplest and most obvious sources of disease vs. health: The food each person decides to eat.

There is no stronger correlation between personal behavior and health outcomes than in the realm of food choice. When a person chooses to eat unhealthful, nutrient-depleted, chemically contaminated processed food, their bodies develop cancer, diabetes, heart disease, Alzheimer's, depression, and other common diseases. But when a person chooses food that's clean, nourishing, and intact, their bodies prevent (and often even reverse) cancer and other serious diseases.

This isn't magic or so-called "woo woo"... it's biochemical cause and effect. Plants produce their own powerful medicines – literally tens of thousands of them – to ward off disease, maximize biological energy, and to adapt and survive in a competitive, stressful ecosystem. When we consume those plants, those same medicines found in plant stems, leaves, nuts, fruits, stalks, and roots often confer similar protective benefits to our own biology. They can suppress "cancer genes," for example, or alter the expression of the genetic code to maximize immune function and prevent infections. These food medicines accelerate healing, normalize blood sugar levels, speed cellular detoxification, invigorate the cardiovascular system, and can even lift a person out of depression.

This book, *Eat to Beat Disease*, tells a simple but powerful truth that every human being needs to hear: Most of us are eating disease promoting foods at every meal. Yet disease preventing foods (and superfoods) are readily available that could replace those toxic foods in the diets of literally billions of people across our planet. The key strategy for human survival, longevity, and the sharp reduction of "sick care" costs is the sharing of knowledge and wisdom about which foods promote rejuvenation and health rather than sickness and disease. This book takes you on a journey of discovery – and sometimes shock – to bring you a wealth of wisdom about how you can transform your health outcomes by changing your day-to-day food choices.

In that way, this book empowers you with personal freedom. On the spectrum of freedom vs. enslavement, there is no worse enslavement than to be a lifelong victim of the for-profit health care system because you ate the disease promoting toxins sold to you by the for-profit junk food industry. Learning to avoid both of these predatory industries grants you an extraordinary sense of personal power, determination, and clarity of thought. In a very real way, learning the knowledge presented in this book will make you a more free person... so much so that the establishment will probably consider you a threat and prefer that you remain nutritionally illiterate and cognitively obedient to the disinformation they often present as "science." But the real science is described in these pages... and the real science says that changing your food choice can not only prevent disease; it can set you free to experience the full joy of human existence that you were meant to experience.

Enjoy the discovery you are about to experience in these pages. Catherine Frompovich set out to write a book about nutrition, detoxification, and food empowerment; but in reality she also wrote a book about freeing people from medical enslavement while uplifting humanity to achieve a greater outcome for us all. It is a journey well worth pursuing.

Mike Adams, the Health Ranger
Editor, NaturalNews.com
Science lab director, CWC Labs
Author, *Food Forensics*

Preface

A man was being chased by a ferocious tiger in the woods, so he ran and he ran until he saw a clearing. He was now up against a cliff's edge, so to escape the tiger, he swung himself over the cliff and began climbing down on a vine. But alas, more tigers awaited him below. He thought he might bide his time and hang on the vine until his predators left, but another predicament then presented itself - two mice came out to chew on the vine and no amount of shooing would make them stop. At this point, he looked around at the face of the cliff and he saw a lone strawberry. In that moment, it was the sweetest strawberry he had ever tasted.

There are many re-tellings of this Zen *koan* and myriad lessons that listeners still derive from it today. If you picked up *Eat to Beat Disease: Foods Medicinal Qualities*, then most likely you are on a healing journey and perhaps even a journey of wisdom. A person today can be easily inundated with lots of conflicting and confusing information about a wide variety of ways to eat and restore his or her health. Some will swear by veganism or vegetarianism; others won't let a meal pass without eating meat. Some say *"carbs" are bad - avoid them like the plague and head toward protein,* while others use carbohydrates for most of their daily intake. Others still will say, *no, fat is what we should have eaten all along.* Go raw and load up on fruit; go cooked and stick with vegetables. Juice - no, blend for the fiber. Which way do you go? What is there to eat?

It's easy to feel more like the man in the Zen story than someone who is confidently strolling down a healing path.

But if we were to compare an individual in this predicament with the man in the Zen story, then perhaps there are a number of other comparisons we could draw with other aspects of the story and those in which find ourselves regarding the food and health situation in our country. Perhaps we could compare the predatory tiger to corporations like Monsanto, Big Food, and Factory Farming - all of which devour a wholesome food supply and run the farmers and consumers into a corner with little choice but to purchase their products. These corporations monopolize, tamper with and lobby themselves into control of the food supply so that consumers must hand their money to them for sustenance instead of being empowered to choose another way. What's found at the bottom of the cliff might be, for the purposes of this example, the regulatory agencies telling the consumer it's safe to go back into the grip of the first tiger.

A consumer, who perceives the revolving door between corporations and government, might grasp at the next solid object to find the way. Perhaps the vine can be likened to hope. It could be a hope in the basic goodness of others to do something to take back their food; for justice to prevail somehow. Or maybe the vine is simply a food and health system in disrepair. This is about the time the consumer is in limbo and is just trying to hang on. Maybe the two mice and the damage they inflict on the vine are comparable to propaganda spread by corporate-sponsored media and science. Their campaigns erode the truth and allow damaging substances to enter the food supply, causing people to throw their hands up and, with apathy, walk away from their health and posterity. All this while the hapless consumer is hanging by a thread, and the chatter of deception is urging him or her to let go; let the rope snap.

What about the strawberry, you wonder. What does it represent? Food invokes the most power over any substance on earth - it means life. Nations rule people by it. We perish without it. It's personal. It is fought about. It can bring us into sweet fellowship. It can heal. It can harm.

This is the milieu in which Catherine Frompovich's book enters. Amidst all of the confusion and the propaganda, Catherine's book provides a compass that allows readers to gather their bearings and gain a direction down the avenues of the power of food and healing. It is a guide that has been greatly needed by all of those who have been attempting to navigate their way through a minefield of misinformation. *Eat to Beat Disease: Foods Medicinal Qualities* is the long awaited conversation about food. Without apology, it repels the establishment lines in ways that other books wouldn't dare.

Heather Callaghan
Editor-in-Chief, *NaturalBlaze.com*

Introduction

Before the latter part of the Industrial Revolution there basically were no man-made toxic chemicals. Chemicals used in growing food crops, food preparation, and processing, or used as flavor enhancers, preservatives, and synthetic ingredients materialized in the 1900s. After World War II, the chemical and pharmaceutical industries began *mentoring* food production. Consequently, there literally are thousands of toxic chemicals that *legally* can be—and are—placed into the food we eat, the water we drink, and the air we breathe. Furthermore, even the U.S. Food and Drug Administration doesn't know what some of those chemicals are thanks to the Toxic Substances Control Act of 1976 loopholes!

What follows is a lose timeline on how the poisoning of agriculture and our food supply came about that we apparently allowed to happen and, even worse, accept!

In 1873, the chemical DDT was first synthesized by a German scientist who didn't appreciate its "value," which Paul Hermann Muller, a Swiss national, finally was able to do in 1939, and for which he was awarded the Nobel Prize for physiology and medicine in 1948. We know what DDT's legacy has been; Rachel Carson told us in her book *Silent Spring*. The National Fertilizer Association was formed in 1883 which, as part of its agenda, was to promote the use of agricultural chemicals.

In 1892, lead arsenate was introduced as a pesticide to control the gypsy moth in the USA. It was the most popular pesticide used in the USA until the 1950s. In 1893, South Carolina phosphate finally became a successful fertilizer selling over 600,000 tons. That, I offer, is the genesis of crop and soil nutrient ruination. Furthermore, the importance of sulfur in farming was endorsed in 1895.

In 1900 there were 6,400,000 farms in the USA. In 2012 there were 3.2 million farmers in the United States—half of what there were 112 years before! Now here is something amazing, I think: 64 percent of all vegetable sales along with 66 percent of all dairy sales come from only 3 percent of large farms or very large family farms, which most likely use chemical soil enhancers and pest controls.

Here's where it gets really interesting: In 1904 the first German chemical cartel was formed. Food adulteration was being recognized for what it was and something was afoot to deal with it: the Pure Food and Drug Act of 1906. It seems the author Upton Sinclair's book *The Jungle* awakened people to what was going on in the then filthy meatpacking industry. Additionally, pesticide poisonings led to public outcry. Why only then and not now, when thousands times more pesticides, chemicals, and other food horrors[2] are happening, especially with regard to one of the most dangerous chemicals ever produced—glyphosate, which is sprayed on food crops like water?

In 1908, it was discovered that pests became resistant to lead arsenate, just sixteen years after its introduction. Can't outsmart those bugs! The same is happening now with genetically modified crops, especially

---

2 http://www.activistpost.com/2014/04/pork-n-pigs.html accessed 2-19-16

corn—the pests, both weeds[3] and insects/worms[4], have become immune or resistant to glyphosate and *Bacillus thuringiensis,* causing huge crop damage and losses.

Here's where the phenomenon of the modern pharmaceutical and chemical industries begins.

> I. *I.G. Farben, the German chemical cartel, forms and includes Bayer, BASF, and Hoechst. I.G. Farben will build chemical plants next to concentration camps during WWII, in support of the Third Reich.*
> II. *Basle A. G., the Swiss chemical cartel, forms to counter I. G. Farben. It includes Ciba, Geigy, and Sandoz. They will dissolve the cartel after World War II but later merge to create Novartus.*[5]

The year 1921 saw the first use of an airplane as a crop duster! In 1924 Rudolph Steiner, founder of the Waldorf Schools, published his book *Agriculture,* the basics of biodynamic agriculture or what some would call organic farming. However, in 1926 Standard Oil (John D Rockefeller 1839-1937) signed a 25 year working agreement [to 1951] with the German cartel, I.G. Farben, the business that would manufacture Adolph Hitler's gas chamber chemicals[6].

The agricultural chemicals' ante is upped big time. In 1928, twenty-nine million pounds of lead arsenate and twenty-nine million pounds of calcium arsenate were applied to food and cotton crops! In 1931 DuPont Chemical Company discovers the pesticidal properties of carbamates whose chemical action is the inhibition of cholinesterase enzymes, which affects nerve impulse transmissions. The very next year, 1932, saw the first use of organophosphates, which have links to adverse

---

3 http://www.ipm.ucdavis.edu/IPMPROJECT/glyphosateresistance.html accessed 2-19-16
4 http://www.wired.com/2014/03/rootworm-resistance-bt-corn/ accessed 2-19-16
5 http://www.chelseagreen.com/blogs/the-history-of-big-chemicals-war-on-food-1865-2007/accessed 2-19-16
6 https://en.wikipedia.org/wiki/Zyklon_B accessed 2-19-16

effects in the neurobehavioral development of fetuses and children—even at low exposure levels!

Organophosphate poisoning is not uncommon; farm workers and families of homes fumigated[7] to treat termites can experience it. I've known of a few people who have been compromised after having their homes treated. In 1933 there were reports of a fifteen-year-old Montana girl poisoned and dying after eating fruit sprayed with arsenic. Methyl bromide[8], a highly toxic fumigant often sprayed on strawberries, was introduced by the California Department of Food and Agriculture in 1936.

In 1927 the U.S. Food and Drug Administration was established, but eleven years later (1938) the Federal Food, Drug, and Cosmetic Act freed the FDA from USDA control by 1940—a really bad move for public safety, in my opinion, and one that has led to the problems we have today with FDA being a virtual extension of the pharmaceutical and chemical industries. Former Monsanto [Roundup® and GMO seeds] chief lobbyist Michael R Taylor, JD, currently is Deputy Commissioner for Foods at the FDA since 2010.

The years 1941 to 1950 saw an agricultural disaster happen to farming—the establishment of monoculture (only one crop) and industrialized farming that depended on using chemicals.

DDT was first used on USA farms in 1945. The very next year, 1946, saw DDT resistance in European houseflies! The animal growth hormone DES for use in U.S. cattle was approved by both the USDA and FDA in 1947. The very next year, 1948, there were reports of

---

7 http://articles.latimes.com/1999/oct/17/realestate/re-23222 accessed 2-19-16
8 http://abcnews.go.com/Health/poisoned-paradise-pesticide-methyl-bromide/story?id=30119220 accessed 2-19-16

DDT resistant houseflies in the U.S. By 1950, houseflies were almost 100 percent resistant to DDT in U.S. dairies!

The saddest thing, I think, that ever came out of a bureaucrat's mouth was what Assistant Secretary of Agriculture Earl Butz (1954) is supposed to have said, [Agriculture] "is now big business" and farmers must "adapt or die."

In 1958 The Delaney Clause became law; it disallowed carcinogenic additives in processed foods. What's happened since? In 1997 President Bill Clinton signed The Food Quality Protection Act of 1996[9] into law that repealed the long-standing Delaney Clause.

Integrated pest management (IPM) was introduced in 1959 and Rachel Carson wrote her best seller book *Silent Spring* in 1962, a clarion awakening to what chemical pesticides were doing to wildlife and human health. In 1965 farm workers/organizers Cesar Chavez and Delores Huerta organized the United Farm Workers to spotlight the harms chemical sprays were doing to food crop workers. I remember those days and promised not to eat grapes, which I did not eat for ten years!

The Environmental Protection Agency (EPA) was established in 1970; it's what I call a "paper tiger" agency—lots of roar but no bite! 1972 saw the suspension of DDT in the USA and the EPA assumed principle authority over pesticides. What good has that done? In 1979 antibiotic- and hormone-treated meat produced in the USA was banned in Europe. But, we still eat it in 2016 in the USA!

This is where food production really becomes "hairy and scary." In 1982 chemical companies pushed support for genetic engineering so that crops could become herbicide resistant. According to reports, by

---

9 http://repository.jmls.edu/cgi/viewcontent.cgi?article=1692&context=lawreview accessed 3-22-16

1984, 447 species of insects were known to be pesticide-resistant while 14 weed species were resistant to one or more herbicides. What does that tell you? Does Nature know how to outwit science?

During 1984, dangerous levels of chlordane/heptachlor were found in milk in six states and its suspension date was made into a "drop dead date of December 31, 1986" with the exception of use for the subsurface treatment of termites. Coincidentally, that same year Israeli female breast cancer rates dropped 30 percent in women below forty-four years of age, just eight years after Israel banned organochlorine pesticides. In 1988 the EPA found 74 different pesticides in 38 agricultural states groundwater.

However, it was not until 1989 that Alar was banned from being sprayed on apples. Actress Meryl Streep became a mom-activist to get Alar off apples. They were successful, and that was the impetus of the demand for organically-grown food in the USA. By 1990, 800,000,000 pounds of pesticides were sprayed on U.S. crops. Two out of five people were expected to contract cancer. The current cancer occurrence rate for U.S. citizens is projected to be one in every two people! I've already had my turn in the cancer barrel, how about you?

The high-water mark year—1994—GMO crops ushered in…

The FDA approves genetically engineered recombinant bovine growth hormone (rBGH or rBST) after a long activist fight. The hormone was developed to increase milk production. The United States already has an enormous surplus of milk.

The genetically engineered Flavr-Savr tomato is approved for sale. It tastes terrible and no one buys it.

Studies link organochlorine chemicals with male reproductive problems and breast cancer. Problems include a 50 percent drop in male sperm count in forty years.

Sales of organic food top two billion dollars. Average sales increases have exceeded 20 percent per year since 1991.

Monsanto and Delta and Pine Land get federal permission to grow genetically modified Roundup Ready cotton. [10]

In 1996 Congress sold out food safety enforcement when it repealed the Delaney Clause!

Food irradiation was approved in 1997 despite 77 percent of Americans being opposed to it. In the mid-1980s, I testified before a U.S. House of Representatives Subcommittee hearing on the dangers of irradiation to foods. I was in opposition to the process and presented reams of scientific information to back my position.

By 1997 these interesting data surfaced regarding herbicides and pesticides in the USA:

- 600+ insects and mites were resistant to one or more pesticides
- 120 weeds were resistant to one or more herbicides
- 115 disease organisms were resistant to pesticides
- 4 million acres of genetically engineered crops were being grown in the USA!

By 1998 the USDA finally proposed organic standards. The organic foods market grows more than 20 percent annually ever since. Is

---

10 http://www.chelseagreen.com/blogs/the-history-of-big-chemicals-war-on-food-1865-2007/ accessed 2-19-16

there any wonder why, when all the poisons that are being sprayed on crops. However, we really don't know if organic crops are free of heavy metals. But, that's a thing of the past because Mike Adams, the Health Ranger who operates the food forensics lab in central Texas since late 2013, has written a book, *Food Forensics*[11], detailing the lab's findings regarding heavy metals in foods, even organically-grown food, which you may want to know about. Adams claims the ICP-MS lab tests confirm that organic foods grown in China cannot be trusted to be heavy-metal-free, as his lab's findings confirm high levels of tungsten[12]. Here's what Mike has to say about that:

> *When I found very high levels of tungsten (greater than 10,000 parts per billion, or ppb) in superfoods imported from China and Southeast Asia, I was told that tungsten was of no concern because "the U.S. Food and Drug Administration (FDA) has no limits on tungsten," and that therefore everyone should ignore the presence of this heavy metal in popular superfood products.* [13]

In 2005 Monsanto accused more than 9,000 farmers of violating its seed patent rules. How can the U.S. Patent Office provide patents for life forms—seeds? Furthermore, those very patents negate Monsanto's and the FDA's claim that GMO foods are the same as non-GMO food. Natural seeds don't carry patents, but GMO seeds do because they have other 'ingredients' in them that natural seeds don't have, e.g., foreign DNA, transgenic[14] and cisgenic[15] proprietary patented "ingredients." By 2007, twelve weeds develop resistance to Monsanto's Roundup®.

---

11 http://www.amazon.com/Food-Forensics-Health-Ranger%C2%92s-Guide/dp/1940363284/ref=sr_1_1?ie=UTF8&qid=1458163831&sr=8-1&keywords=food+forensics
12 Mike Adams, Food Forensics, (Dallas, TX: BenBellaBooks, 2016), Pg. 2.
13 Ibid.
14 http://www.thefreedictionary.com/transgenic accessed 3-4-16
15 http://www.cisgenesis.com/content/view/2/25/lang,english/ accessed 3-4-16

According to published statistics, 2.6 billion pounds of Monsanto's glyphosate (Roundup®) were sprayed on U.S. agricultural lands between 1992 and 2012!

The total amount of fertilizer applied in fiscal year 2008, according to The Fertilizer Institute, was "54.9 million tons of material...in the United States." Moreover, I found something I thought was rather humorous on the institute's website regarding which countries use and produce the most fertilizers: "*The largest consuming countries are generally those with the larger populations and those with the best diets. They are: China, India, the United States and Brazil.*" Best diets in USA? Then why did I feel compelled to write this book? Let's see how those four countries rate in health statistics.

According to the Commonwealth Fund Overall Country Rankings[16], of the four countries listed above, the only one I found was the USA, and it ranked last of the eleven countries listed: Australia, Canada, France, Germany, Netherlands, New Zealand, Norway, Sweden, Switzerland, the UK, and the USA.

One of the categories listed for all countries is "Healthy Lives" and the USA came in at number 11, the last, spending an average—and the highest per capita amount—of $8,508 for health expenditures for the year 2011. Last! Shouldn't the USA be first, if it is supposed to have a "best diet." France came in at number 1 in healthy lives; Sweden, number 2; Switzerland, 3; Australia, 4; Netherlands, 5; Norway, 6; Germany, 7; Canada, 8; New Zealand, 9; the UK, 10; and the USA, 11.

Now, here's where it really gets interesting—"World Health Organization Ranking; the World's Health Systems"[17] lists the ratings of 190 countries. China is ranked 144; India, 112; Brazil, 125; and

---

16 http://www.commonwealthfund.org/publications/press-releases/2014/jun/us-health-system-ranks-last accessed 2-19-16

17 http://thepatientfactor.com/canadian-health-care-information/world-health-organizations-ranking-of-the-worlds-health-systems/ accessed 2-19-16

USA, 37. You would think if those countries had the "best diets," they'd have better health systems. Morocco at 29 is ahead of the USA! I was in Morocco and I can tell you the food there truly is locally farmed, especially the foods the Berbers, who traditionally have been farmers, bring in from the countryside.

My late husband used to remind me of a cultural saying he heard as a child that translates to "Good health begins in the cook pot." They had that right, I say.

Furthermore, in the early 20th century, two perceptive health researchers and practitioners, Dr Weston A Price, DDS (1870-1948) and Dr Francis M Pottenger Jr, MD (1901-1967) began "to beat the drums" about proper nutrition and how its implementation, or lack thereof, would affect human health. Dr Price did exceptional research around the globe regarding the status of dental and overall health as correlated with diets. What he found truly was amazing:

> *"The isolated people Price photographed—with their fine bodies, ease of reproduction, emotional stability and freedom from degenerative ills—stand in sharp contrast to civilized moderns subsisting on the 'displacing foods of modern commerce,' including sugar, white flour, pasteurized milk, lowfat foods, vegetable oils and convenience items filled with extenders and additives."* [18]

Dr Price found that the degeneration process in cats was "complete" after only three generations; whereas in rats, it took eight generations of eating degenerated diets. Price is remembered as saying something to the effect that in each generation eating a degenerational diet, there is a progressive degeneration of the species. He surmised that was happening in humans because of societal degeneration, plus the emergence of

---

18 http://www.westonaprice.org/health-topics/abcs-of-nutrition/principles-of-healthy-diets-2/ accessed 3-8-16

type 2 diabetes, cancers, and heart disease. Many more diseases—some of which were not on medicine's radar, e.g., HIV/AIDS for example—have become commonplace and chronic since both doctors did their remarkable research.

According to the World Health Organization, the top ten leading causes of death according to a 2012 report are categorized according to low income countries, lower middle income countries, upper middle income countries, and high income countries.[19] Interestingly, Alzheimer's and breast cancer appear in the statistics for high income countries. Cancer statistics appear only in the upper middle income and high income countries.

I want to express my sincere thanks to Chelsea Green Publishing Blog for their exceptional "History of Big Chemical's War on Food, 1865—2007" that enabled me to extrapolate and create a semblance of a timeline so you can get an idea of what's been going on for decades regarding food which, unfortunately, has become a "political football" that, literally, impacts our health and wellbeing.

Also, a word of thanks to Mike Adams, author of the 2016 book, *Food Forensics*, for his commitment to exposing the hidden and negative side of food ingredients, which manufacturers apparently don't want us to know about, since it's not listed on ingredient labels. Here are some of his lab's remarkable findings:

In just the first few months of ICP-MS research on samples of foods, vitamins, and consumer products, I discovered:

- *More than 500 ppb mercury in cat treats and fish-based dog treats*
- *More than 10 ppm tungsten in rice protein products*

---

19 http://www.who.int/mediacentre/factsheets/fs310/en/index1.html accessed 3-8-16

- *More than 5 ppm lead [Pb] in ginkgo herb products*
- *More than 11 ppm lead in mangosteen powder*
- *More than 400 ppb lead in cacao powders*
- *More than 500 ppb lead and more than 2,000 ppb cadmium in rice proteins*
- *More than 6 ppm arsenic and more than 1 ppm lead in some spirulina products*
- *More than 500 ppb mercury in dog treats*
- *More than 200 ppb lead in brand-name mascara products*

(Note: 1,000 ppb = 1 ppm)

In nearly every case, when I contacted the manufacturer of the product to warn them about the high levels of heavy metals found in their products, they insisted their products were perfectly safe while urging me to remain silent and keep their secret from the public.[20]

That fact alone, I think, ought to be incentive enough that everyone would want to eat as nutritiously and toxin-free as possible. I truly was impressed with Mike Adams' exceptional book and encourage you to check it out, as it really complements what you will read in this book.

This book, nevertheless, does not begin to cover all the varied aspects and sciences of food, nutrition, diet, plus ensuing health consequences. What I've tried to do is whet your appetite about what real food, especially plant-based nutrition, can do to improve your health and wellbeing. For each topic I discuss, I could write a separate book just about that. However, I feel I've addressed what I think are issues affecting most people, which you probably don't know, and how you can get started on the road to claiming and maintaining better health just by what you put, or don't put, into your mouth.

---

20 Mike Adams, *Food Forensics,* (Dallas, TX: BenBellaBooks, 2016), Pp.3-4.

My belief is you can't poison a body into wellness, and you have to "eat to beat disease."

Catherine J Frompovich
April 2016

What's the Premise Behind "There's a science to eating?"

*W*hat is the rationale for a book about eating to gain health and overcoming disease using food and dietary choices plus sound eating habits? *"Eat to beat disease!"* It really is a matter of scientific fact that an inadequate diet can weaken one's resistance to disease. The immune system is the safeguard of human health.

As I perceive, *fusion-style cuisine* probably is familiar to most folks, and it's extremely popular on the restaurant scene. Although, the term is a comparatively recent (1970s) minted epicurean classification for combining elements of different ethnic and culinary traditions into today's modern restaurant menus, it's appeal is that it offers exciting variety and tastes that utilize an eclectic approach to food preparation, restaurant fare, and fine dining.

Similarly, my approach to health-regeneration in this book is with food facts, science, and sample recipes to bring a similar fusion-like creativity to "eat to beat disease" that not only will turn on taste buds, but also entice and enable molecular biochemistry to prove unequivocally what Hippocrates, the Father of Modern Medicine, sagaciously advised so very long ago, *"Let medicine be thy food, and food be thy medicine."*

First and foremost, this book is offered in the hope of helping readers understand the varied nutritional reasons for eating in a manner so as to "eat to beat disease." Hopefully, readers will welcome an opportunity to take charge of their health, not feel overwhelmed, or at a loss as to why changes in eating patterns undoubtedly will have to be made—some rather drastically—especially if you are a "junk food addict."

Societies that survive on the modern western diet of fast foods, diet sodas, sugar-laden snacks, and fatty red meats, actually eat their way to health problems and disease. The resulting state of *dis-ease* unequivocally stems from avoiding ample amounts of fiber and fresh, nutrient-rich, plant-based foods such as vegetables, nuts, seeds, and fruit, while opting instead for highly-processed and chemicalized foodstuffs.

Numerous studies confirm when individuals change from their traditional or ethnic diets, e.g., the Japanese and most Asians, to the modern U.S. fast food diet, health demographics change dramatically and correspondingly to mirror disease patterns in western civilizations where junk foods are main dietary staples. How unfortunate! Cancer and heart disease rates confirm there's a common denominator; it's the lack of sound and healthful, nutritional, fresh food dietary practices.

The U.S./modern western diet is based in fast foods, sugar-laden edibles with highly chemicalized and synthetic ingredients. Instead of real, whole food ingredients, it's cost effective and significantly cheaper to use chemicals that mimic vegetable flavors leaving very little nutritional content and fiber, all while adding insidious disproportionate amounts of salt and chemical residues to human body tissues and organs, which, obviously, lead to toxicity, inflammation, and chronic diseases.

Plant-based foods contain a wealth of elements – fiber, vitamins, minerals, enzymes, antioxidants, even plant proteins – which actually become the fuel or building blocks of the life energy force ATP (Adenosine triphosphate)[21] for all human cell mitochondria. That biochemical fact needs to be considered seriously, if not studied, in order to appreciate fully that you cannot feed a body processed and junk foods, plus chemicals, which are in just about everything, and expect to be healthy.

I used to tell my nutrition clients, "You can't poison a body into wellness."

An excellent analogy about an organism requiring proper fuel to run can be your car. You cannot put sugar into a car's gas tank and expect the car to run. Or water! An automobile, which is a piece of machinery, knows what it needs to operate, but many humans still can't understand the importance of eating nutritiously to avoid disease.

Besides that, there's a nutritional myth about protein. Many, if not most, people think that protein is the most important food to eat, so they over-indulge, not knowing that animal proteins can be problematic disease factors for various reasons. Food animals are fed antibiotics to gain weight, plus GMO crops like alfalfa, corn, and soy, which leave toxic residues in their milk and meat, plus toxins are found as residues in their products and also in humans who eat them.

Animal protein can be detrimental to health when, as in the modern American diet, too much animal protein is eaten, e.g., a 12-ounce Porterhouse steak served eaten with a baked potato smothered in dairy

---

21 https://en.wikipedia.org/wiki/Adenosine_triphosphate accessed 11/16/15

sour cream, then topped off with a chocolate ice cream sundae for dessert. Too much protein[22] in the diet can cause purines to form along with high levels of uric acid, causing gout, or contribute to kidney stones[23] or kidney diseases such as Proteinuria.

Enzymes, especially those plant-based food enzymes eaten as raw foods, act like miniature keys that unlock cell doors so micro nutrients can become bioavailable for body chemistry. Consequently, previously nutritionally-stressed or deprived cells eventually become enlivened, or rejuvenated, by raw food enzymes. Furthermore, enzymes help our bodies break down food micronutrients, which are essential to every cell in our bodies. Are you aware that you are as healthy as your sickliest cell—and that your body has anywhere from 37 to 50 trillion cells? Are you aware that you have a huge crowd to feed and keep well on a daily basis?

When diets lack full-spectrum natural nutrition, certain vitamin deficiency diseases can and do occur, such as Beriberi (lack of B-1), Ariboflavinosis (lack of B-2), Pellagra (lack of B-3) and numerous other diseases[24] that you ought to become familiar with in order to understand the importance of proper nutritional eating habits, which is one of the goals of this book. "Eat to beat disease" realistically means maximum nutrient content affecting biochemistry enhancement with every morsel we put into our mouths. Hopefully, you find this book to be "user friendly" and a helpful resource, which can enable you to accomplish your goal: "eat to beat disease."

As an author, I get it that most folks don't like having to read through an inordinate amount of information to get what they need or want.

---

22 http://www.ncbi.nlm.nih.gov/pmc/articles/PMC1262767/ accessed 11-16-15
23 http://www.mayoclinic.org/diseases-conditions/kidney-stones/basics/causes/con-20024829 accessed 11-16-15
24 http://www.healthsupplementsnutritionalguide.com/vitamin-deficiency-symptoms.html accessed 11-16-15

That being said, I hope my readers will consider this a "meat and potatoes" type book, even though it addresses health from *a fusion diet* approach, featuring more plant-based foods, organically grown, which are naturally-packed with all the inherent nutrients needed to regulate body chemistry. I know of people who have un-grown tumors; nutritionally induced cancer-cell apoptosis (cell suicide); and restored vibrant health without surgery, chemotherapy, or radiation. I am one of those people—a breast cancer survivor.

Probably, the most important—and first—aspect of eating nutriously is to restructure your food buying habits to exclude junk foods, processed foods, sugar treats and candies, and to purchase organically-grown whole foods: vegetables, fruits, nuts, seeds, and as many other foods—including an occasional treat—organically-grown. I also suggest purchasing food that is locally-grown. Consumers need to support local farmers and co-operatives, as they are the *real food* growers—not big corporate agriculture.

Personally, I've noticed a huge taste difference in local-to-my-region (Ambler, PA) grown broccoli as compared with California-grown broccoli. Even the young man, who works in the produce department of one of the stores I frequent, expressed the same comment, which I thought was very perceptive of him. So, here's the long and short of locally-grown food: Different soil mineral content determines taste and nutrients; fresher quality with much less travel time affecting less nutrient degradation; and the pride in knowing you're keeping farmers in your region growing healthful food. I think farmers are the most important people in any economy.

Not only is organically-grown food nutrient content higher[25] and actually tastes better, but organically-grown crops cannot be sprayed

---

25 http://www.npr.org/sections/thesalt/2014/07/11/330760923/are-organic-vegetables-more-nutritious-after-all accessed 11-17-15

with toxic pesticides and herbicides that are harmful to human health, nor can they be genetically modified, or subjected to certain food processes like food irradiation. Many brand-name herbs and spices are irradiated[26].

Having said all the above, may I introduce you to several studies that talk about organically-grown food being *nutrient-rich*? One is "Nutritional Quality of Organic Versus Conventional Fruits, Vegetables, and Grains"[27] and the other, "Fruit and Soil Quality of Organic and Conventional Strawberry Agroecosystems"[28]. Another is "Higher antioxidant and lower cadmium concentrations and lower incidence of pesticide residues in organically grown crops: a systematic literature review and meta-analyses"[29], which emphasizes the importance of the lack of pesticides and heavy metal residues, while emphasizing higher antioxidant content and values—keys to healthful eating.

Sustainable farmer Joel Salatin, of Polyface Farms in rural Virginia, quips, "If you think organic food is expensive, have you priced cancer lately?"

Just to impress upon you how profitable sickness really is for those who try to manage it, rather than really cure diseases, e.g., the pharmaceutical industry, diabetes alone is a billion-dollar-a-year business!

The Alzheimer's Association estimates that the costs associated with Alzheimer's will be a TRILLION U.S. dollars by 2050.

---

26 https://www.organicconsumers.org/old_articles/Irrad/irradfact.php accessed 1-13-2016
27 http://journeytoforever.org/farm_library/worthington-organic.pdf accessed 11-16-15
28 http://journals.plos.org/plosone/article?id=10.1371/journal.pone.0012346 accessed 11-16-15
29 http://journals.cambridge.org/action/displayAbstract;jsessionid=909EDF7D4F6602450520DCDD5E829301.journals?aid=9325471&fileId=S0007114514001366 accessed 11-16-15

In January 2016, I wrote the article "Are You Aware of Big Pharma's Impressive Records?" [30] wherein I cited the death statistics for numerous pharmaceutical drugs from January 1, 2000. Chemotherapy drug deaths totaled 16,043,519!

Regarding cancer, the total of all health care costs for treating cancers in the USA for 2011 only, were $88.7 Billion![31]

With such revenue stream capabilities, why would any business want to find a cure for a disease or health problem that would reduce its profits? However and to the contrary, patients who suffer with chronic diseases get impacted in countless ways, but the most personal and direct include being sick, tired, worn out, in pain, disabled, or just plain distraught at not finding or attaining wellness.

Statistical proof, of sorts, to back up that last comment can be found in the fact that, according to a *Journal of the American Medical Association (JAMA)* November 2015 article, "Trends in Prescription Drug Use Among Adults in the United States From 1999 – 2012," *"The prevalence of polypharmacy…increased from an estimated 8.2% in 1999-2000 to 15% in 2011-12…"*[32] That's almost double! Polypharmacy, by the way, is the use of multiple pharmaceutical drugs by one person.

Numerous senior citizens take as high as five or more prescription drugs *daily*![33-34] That, unfortunately in my opinion, is testimony to a dietary and lifestyle nutritionally deficient and probably based in fast-

---

30   http://www.activistpost.com/2016/01/are-you-aware-of-big-pharmas-impressive-records.html accessed 1-14-2016
31   http://www.cancer.org/cancer/cancerbasics/economic-impact-of-cancer accessed 11-18-15
32   http://jama.jamanetwork.com/article.aspx?articleid=2467552 accessed 11-19-15
33   http://www.prnewswire.com/news-releases/new-survey-shows-seniors-struggle-under-the-weight-of-multiple-medication-use-80246652.html accessed 12-15-15
34   https://www.cihi.ca/en/types-of-care/pharmaceutical-care-and-utilization/most-seniors-take-5-or-more-drugs-numbers-double accessed 12-15-15

food convenience and chain restaurants, packaged and processed starchy carbohydrates, and snacking foods, while foregoing "scratch cooking" that uses nutrient-rich, plant-based, whole foods grown organically.

As a western culture, we've gotten into convenience eating full-time, rather than healthful eating. There's even a meme making the rounds that folks who exercise due diligence about eating nutritiously are psych cases. They've coined medical terminology for the 'problem'; it's "orthorexia". Would you believe that eating healthfully is now considered a mental and psychiatric disorder? [35]

However, as one who earned her degrees in *natural* nutrition and holistic health sciences in the 1970s and 1980s, I have to wonder what happened during the ensuing years so that the nutrition information I learned back then, only recently has become vogue-like information in every magazine and the media with allopathic medical doctors, who learned virtually nothing about nutrition in med schools, even jumping on board the nutrition bandwagon. Don't you hear them giving food and nutrition advice on radio and television?

The ironic part about medical doctors and nutrition, for me at least, is that I remember as late as the 1980s, one medical doctor, who was head of a pediatric hospital, saying to me, "If there was anything to nutrition, wouldn't you think we'd know about it?"

Currently with such a super-saturated culture of foodies, organically-grown foods and wines, sustainable agriculture, vegetarian and vegan restaurants, gluten-free menus, Paleo, raw foods and other diets, one has to wonder how come it has taken so long to reach this degree of food consciousness, and still it's considered a mental or psychiatric disorder to want—and eat—nutritiously. Duh!

---

35 http://naturalsociety.com/officials-declare-eating-healthy-mental-disorder/ accessed 12-15-15

With all the above going on, however, I think there still is a need for a book like this. Why do I say that? Because often it is confusing, and even complicated, trying to regain or maintain health, especially when more lip service is given to the need for and implementation of a healthful dietary and lifestyle than there are ways and means to secure and implement the information and obtain long-sought-after results.

In spring of 2013, Kaiser Permanente, the largest managed healthcare system, published in *The Permanente Journal* the paper "Nutritional Update for Physicians: Plant-based Diets"[36] wherein the Abstract, this most apparent "*counter orthorexia statement*" held:

> *"Concerns about the rising cost of health care are being voiced nationwide, even as unhealthy lifestyles are contributing to the spread of obesity, diabetes, and cardiovascular disease. For these reasons, physicians looking for cost-effective interventions to improve health outcomes are becoming more involved in helping their patients adopt healthier lifestyles. Healthy eating may be best achieved with a plant-based diet, which we define as a regimen that encourages whole, plant-based foods and discourages meats, dairy products, and eggs as well as all refined and processed foods. We present a case study as an example of the potential health benefits of such a diet."*

Furthermore, that article went on to say plant-based diets are cost effective; reduce the number of medications that are needed to treat chronic diseases; and physicians should consider recommending plant-based diets to their high blood pressure, diabetes, cardiovascular disease, and obesity patients. Wow! What validation for this book.

---

[36] http://www.thepermanentejournal.org/issues/2013/spring/5117-nutrition.html accessed 12-16-15

As an added segue, I'd like to interject at this introductory phase in the book that the late Max Gerson, MD, (1881-1959)[37] a pioneer in holistic cancer treatment who founded the Gerson Therapy, which uses a strict plant-based dietary approach, realized that when his cancer patients were cured but returned to their meat-and-animal-products-diets, cancers returned! However, when those same patients went back on Dr Gerson's plant-based protocol, the cancers and tumors went into remission. That happened too often, thereby prompting Dr Gerson to "connect the dots" regarding diet, food, and disease, especially cancer. Nevertheless, Dr Gerson's work is not respected by allopathic medicine and the chemotherapy-based, pharmaceutical multi-billion-dollar-a-year cancer industry[38]. A stunning and rather ironic aspect of six of the chemotherapy drugs listed in footnote 38, which are annotated with a star, states

> *"The drugs marked with a* [5-point-star icon] *are listed in the "11th Report of Carcinogens" of the US National Toxicology Program as "carcinogenic", i.e. cancer causing. In other words, the drugs prescribed to millions of cancer patients as a cure, are in fact, known to cause cancer."*

Personally, I feel Dr Gerson was so ahead of the curve on health and healing in using food and nutrition that his work had to be discounted for obvious peer-pressure control and financial reasons. I conjecture that academic/professional rejection, plus castigation, resulted from Dr Gerson's totally natural, dietary, non-pharmaceutical, non-chemo-radiation-based approach to managing and curing disease, especially cancer, which is the mega-money maker for oncologists and pharmaceutical companies.

---

37 http://www.amazon.com/Dr-Max-Gerson-Healing-Hopeless/dp/155082290X accessed 12-16-15
38 http://www.chemo-facts.com/ accessed 12-16-15

However, there is the human need for "comfort food," satiety and what's called "umami"—those food ingredients that make foods satisfying. For most adults, umami includes the taste and the sensory feel of meats and fats not only in the mouth, but after digestion—a sated satisfaction; whereas, children prefer sugar and starches. The four tastes we consciously recognize are salty, sweet, bitter, and sour. A fifth sensory perception regarding food is "umami," a Japanese word, which incorporates the emotional and physical aspects of what makes foods satisfying to each individual.

For those who want to maintain a strict plant-based diet, umami can be elusive at times, since most fatty foods, especially those from animal sources, are not included in the dietary. Fat and salt contribute to satiety and umami. To accomplish plant-based food umami, I suggest including avocados, olives, nut butters, cold-pressed oils, toasted sesame oil, toasted sesame seeds, raw sunflower seeds, and chopped nuts as garnish along with sliced scallions, and cooking with onions, medicinal mushrooms—some, like Maitake and French horn, have the tactile feel of meat in the mouth, tomatoes or tomato sauce, miso, tempeh, and Braggs Amino Acids.

One satisfying dietary "trick" when you are not satisfied after eating and you feel you need something sweet, is to eat a handful of raw pecans or walnuts. Instantaneously, you will feel satisfied and have no craving for something sweet like dessert.

Freshly squeezed lemon or lime juice always adds some zing to any dish, I think, plus it turns into an alkaline ash during digestion. Include some lemon zest in your cooking too. Personally, I don't approve of vinegar in the diet—it's highly acidic and actually can be 'addictive', especially balsamic vinegar. We find vinegar in condiments like catsup, horseradish, mayonnaise, mustard, pickles, relishes plus sweet 'n sour dishes—all highly satisfying to the taste buds. However, the wide-ranging idea of eating for health is to eat as much of an alkaline ash base diet as possible. Vinegar is very acidic, ranging between a 2 to 2.4 pH on the acid/alkaline balance scale. Some apple cider vinegars advertise a pH of 3.075, still in the acidic range. Seven is neutral, whereas anything over 7 is considered alkaline.

There are innumerable benefits to eating a plant-based, alkaline ash diet. The addition of fresh fruits, greens, and vegetables—most of which are alkaline base—definitely improves the Potassium/Sodium balance in the body. Potassium is to soft body tissue what calcium is to bone. Improving the K/Na balance benefits the bones and reduces chronic diseases such as hypertension, heart disease, and stroke. Since most fruits and vegetables are excellent sources of magnesium, all enzyme systems would benefit greatly, especially the utilization of vitamin D.

Magnesium lowers diabetes risk, increases mental clarity, and reduces anxiety and depression.

Resources

Astounding Number of Medical Procedures Have No Benefit, Even Harm – JAMA Study
http://www.thesleuthjournal.com/astounding-number-of-medical-procedures-have-no-benefit-even-harm-jama-study/accessed 11-16-15

Update on Medical Practices That Should Be Questioned in 2015
http://archinte.jamanetwork.com/article.aspx?articleid=2469079 accessed 11-16-15

What's the Cause of Most Diseases?

Rather than bore readers with my hypothesis regarding the causes of disease, I think nothing could state it better—or be more convincing—than what a team of research scientists at Stony Brook University (New York) found and went public with December 16, 2015 in their article "Substantial contribution of intrinsic risk factors to cancer development" published in the journal *Nature*[39].

Four researchers, Scott Powers, Yusuf Hannun, Song Wu and Wei Zhu, concluded, as per the Abstract,

"Collectively, we conclude that cancer risk is heavily influenced by extrinsic factors. These results are important for strategizing cancer prevention, research and public health." They estimated that up to 90 percent of all cancers are caused environmentally, e.g., chemicals and their outgassing, residues, and contamination of air, water, food, cosmetics, clothing, furniture, mattresses—you name it!

Furthermore, in my 2009 book *Our Chemical Lives And The Hijacking Of Our DNA, A Probe Into What's Probably Making Us Sick*, I discussed in great length (over 400 pages) what chemicals do to our body's systems and DNA. For anyone interested in reading that definitive book, it's available on Amazon.com.

---

39 http://www.nature.com/nature/journal/vaop/ncurrent/full/nature16166.html accessed 12-24-15

More and more, research, science, and medicine are pointing to epigenetics as a principle co-factor in disease. What is epigenetics, you probably are asking? According to *Wikipedia,* it's *"cellular and physiological phenotypic trait variations that are caused by external or environmental factors that switch genes on and off and affect how cells read genes instead of being caused by changes in the DNA sequence."*

And what are those external or environmental factors? The answer, unequivocally, is chemicals of all types: agricultural, industrial, and medical—including pharmaceuticals and vaccines; man-made environmental pollution from innumerable causes—especially weather geoengineering chemtrails[40]; radiation; and electromagnetic frequencies in various ranges, namely microwaves from cell phones and towers, Wi-Fi, utilities AMI smart meters, and microwave ovens; plus some naturally-occurring toxins found in Nature, e.g., Arctic methane[41]. Methane usually contains non-toxic and toxic gases—one being carbon monoxide. And, you can add medical malpractice mistakes, e.g., the over-prescribing of prescription drugs, especially psychotropic meds.

---

40 http://stopsprayingcalifornia.com/ accessed 12-24-15
41 http://onlinelibrary.wiley.com/doi/10.1002/2015GL065013/abstract accessed 12-24-15

What's Trending Health-wise with Baby-boomers?

Everyone is familiar with trends, especially trending on the Internet. Well, there's something that's trending, but not boding well, for younger Americans aged 15 to 44. Medically, it's called cerebrovascular accident, which commonly is referred to as a stroke. The incident rate in that age group has risen by 53 percent, while the incidence rate for the general population under 65 years of age has risen from 25 to 31 percent.

But what is even more startling is the fact that about 80 percent of strokes can be prevented.

Knowing your risk factors and blood pressure readings, along with not smoking, probably are the first line of prevention. The other preventable factor is proper weight/body mass for your gender, age, and height. Obesity definitely is another factor in upping the trend toward rising stroke rates.

Diet and food are the main tools for preventing strokes and also for weight control. Many physicians advise salt restriction, which really can be confusing and even difficult to achieve, since most salt intake is in the form of hidden sodium in chemicals used in processed/packaged foods, snacks, restaurants, and fast food outlets.

Sodium (salt) actually is an important mineral the body needs for life, since it's one of the major electrolytes in human body chemistry. There are four minerals that make up the major electrolytes: sodium, potassium, magnesium, and chloride. When people become dehydrated, especially the elderly, they have to be hooked up to an intravenous (IV) drip to rehydrate them. In that drip are sodium, potassium, sterile water, and other supplementation needed at the time.

Sodium gets a bum rap insofar as we are told to eliminate it, when we actually need it for life. Sodium is important for the electrical signals in the body, which allow our muscles and brain to work. Actually, it's half of the "electrical pump" at cellular level that keeps sodium in the plasma (yellow liquid component of human blood) and potassium inside the cell! See how important sodium really is.

Many doctors are now rethinking the role of salt/sodium in managing high blood pressure, which means that HBP patients can use table salt sparingly. However, processed table salt is not ideal salt to put into a salt shaker, I offer. It contains sugar (sucrose) and free-flowing chemicals, which you don't need. Those ingredients take away from the salty taste, so you sprinkle a lot more salt, I offer.

I contend that vegetables, pastas, rice, etc., should not be cooked in salted water. Use salt sparingly while preparing food. Learn how to use organically-grown fresh and dried herbs for taste. Then you can allow each person to sprinkle either sea salt or preferably Himalaya pink salt (an ancient sea salt now mined on land) on to his/her food at table. Pink salt definitely tastes more salty than processed table salt and even sea salt, I contend, so you tend to use quite a bit *less* salt to defeat any flat taste of food.

Salt is found in high quantities in pickles, olives, chips, munchies, cured meats, packaged condiments and spreads, popcorn, snack and fast foods, cereals, sodas including sugar-free, canned foods, and even some cheeses. I suggest always buying salt-free foods, e.g., rice cakes, peanut butter, butter, etc. Here's [42] an online shopper's guide to finding lower sodium foods in supermarkets.

A few years ago, I wrote the article "Don't Have Faulty Ideas About Salt" for *Easy Health Options* [43] in which I said the following:

1. The average American eats between 4,000 and 6,000 mg of sodium/salt a day.
2. There are subtle differences between plant-based sodium and table salt that the medical and pharmaceutical industries and health agencies don't make clear to consumers. Said differences influence whether body chemistry works efficiently or detrimentally.
3. Contrast this unbalanced emphasis on sodium to the mineral balance in vegetables. Fresh asparagus, which is a great aid to kidney health, contains almost six times as much potassium as sodium. Bananas are also rich in potassium. Nature embedded various nutrients within all plant foods that automatically balance nutrient status if and when we eat a varied diet of organically grown food, as raw or unprocessed as possible, without chemicals or genetically modified organisms.
4. Conventional medicine is trying to pigeonhole everyone's sodium/potassium ratios into a one-size-fits-all model that overprescribes blood pressure medications. But these medications may be doing more harm than good, by taking minerals out of the body and harming the kidneys.
5. An imbalance in sodium and potassium may also be responsible for heart arrhythmias or, perhaps, dementias linked to strong diuretics that drain the body of fluids and essential nutrients. And too many people forget to drink plenty of pure water.

---

42 http://www.dietitiancenter.com/article.aspx?id=12 accessed 1-10-2016
43 http://easyhealthoptions.com/dont-have-faulty-ideas-about-salt/ accessed 1-10-2016

Here are some comparative examples of *processed food salt contents* compared with *naturally-occurring sodium levels* in plant-based foods:

One cup drained snap green beans canned	354 mg sodium [mostly NaCl]
One cup cooked without salt fresh green beans	1 mg [natural-occurring] sodium
One cup drained broccoli cooked without salt	64 mg [natural-occurring] sodium
One tablespoon salted butter	82 mg sodium [mostly NaCl]
One tablespoon unsalted butter	2 mg [natural-occurring] sodium
12 ounces carbonated ginger ale soda	26 mg sodium
One cup drained carrots canned	353 mg sodium [mostly NaCl]
One cup drained cooked fresh carrots	90 mg [natural-occurring] sodium

NaCl is Sodium Chloride, common table salt or halite. Salt actually acts as a binder in sausage making and also as a tenderizer. Salt also is considered and used as a preservative that inhibits the growth of bacteria. Some people may experience "salt burns" on their tongues from eating very salty foods. Has that ever happened to you? Too much salt also can lead to digestive problems.

Everything has to be in balance, including the proper use of salt in the diet.

Another health problem that can be considered as trending, in my opinion, is metabolic syndrome, which is characterized by obesity, hypertension, and other dysfunctional metabolic issues that can lead to risks of diabetes, heart attack, stroke, dementia, kidney disease, and fatty liver. Nearly 50 percent of U.S. citizens over 40 years of age have metabolic syndrome! If you have a "pot belly," and especially if you are male, you ought to explore metabolic syndrome.

Incidentally, most metabolic syndrome cases start out with insulin resistance, which usually results from nutritionally poor diets like those based in fast food chain menus and starchy carbohydrates (pizza, pasta, pastries, and chips) guzzled down with beer or soda.

Obesity doesn't say a body is well fed; to the contrary, it indicates a body that is malnourished. The most effective treatment for dealing with metabolic syndrome is diet and exercise, as documented in an article in *Journal of Applied Physiology*[44].

However, in a 2016 article published in the *Journal of Nutrition*, aged garlic extract had been shown to reverse plaque in arteries and to prevent the progression of heart disease. That's a clue, I think, about the importance of using plenty of fresh garlic in cooking and your diet. Garlic also is known to help prevent cancer and other chronic diseases associated with ageing!

Furthermore, Nathan Pritikin proved that a diet high in plant-based foods containing unrefined veggies, beans, whole grains, and fruits—plus exercise—not only could reverse heart disease, but would prevent it. Pritikin co-authored the 1979 book, *The Pritikin Program for Diet and Exercise*, which became a *New York Times* best seller.

---

44   http://jap.physiology.org/content/100/5/1657 accessed 1-22-16

Other men of science and medicine have gone on to champion the role of diet and nutrition in the etiology, cure, and prevention of disease: Neal D Barnard, MD; T. Colin Campbell, PhD; John A McDougall, MD; and Dean Ornish, MD—just to name a few.

So you see how important a plant-based diet is for regaining and also maintaining optimum health.

However, those under forty years of age[45] are experiencing colorectal[46] and gastrointestinal cancers at an increasingly much higher rate, which health researchers think is attributed to their poor diets and food choices. Forsaking nutrient- and fiber-filled plant foods for fast food menus of burgers, fries, pizza, and high carbohydrate snack foods eventually takes its toll health wise.

In the May 2015 published report "Rising Rates of Sporadic Colorectal Cancer in Young Adults: A Possible Environmental Link," the author Monica Malik, MD, says, *"The traditional Indian diet, consisting predominantly of plant-based, fiber-rich foods and antioxidant-rich spices, has been postulated to be protective."*[47] Dr Malik is right on, I contend. Plant-based, fiber-rich diets offer more nutrients for attaining and maintaining optimum health than the "fast food generation" may realize.

It is my hope that *Eat to Beat Disease* becomes encouragement to explore healthful food choices.

---

45 http://www.nytimes.com/2007/01/30/health/30canc.html?_r=0 accessed 3-12-16
46 http://am.asco.org/rising-rates-sporadic-colorectal-cancer-young-adults-possible-environmental-link accessed 3-12-16
47 Ibid.

What Goes In Must Come Out: A necessary discussion about poop

---

This is going to be an extremely delicate topic to discuss, so I will make it as easy, and sanitized, as possible. However, it is the counterbalancing information to all that is said about eating food, nutrition, and how we can 'read' tell-tale 'cryptograms' of sorts, as to how food is being utilized and evacuated from our bodies.

Attaining a healthful and nutritional life status includes the following: purchasing and correctly preparing nutrient-rich, organically-grown foods, *which are digested, assimilated, and eliminated effectively for biosynthesis. That* is the *real* secret to nutritional success, so please take seriously what's said in this chapter about what your poop may be telling you.

Below is the *Bristol Stool Chart*[48], which depicts 7 types of stool a normal human body can produce. Only one, in my opinion, is the ideal specimen; it is Type 4: sausage or snake like, and smooth as toothpaste. One of the physicians I know refers to that ideal specimen as an "FLF"—foot-long-floater!

---

48   Google Bristol Stool Chart accessed online 3-4-16

Bristol Stool Chart

Type 1		Separate hard lumps, like nuts (hard to pass)
Type 2		Sausage-shaped but lumpy
Type 3		Like a sausage but with cracks on the surface
Type 4		Like a sausage or snake, smooth and soft
Type 5		Soft blobs with clear-cut edges
Type 6		Fluffy pieces with ragged edges, a mushy stool
Type 7		Watery, no solid pieces. Entirely Liquid

Analyzing what exits the body as poop takes some getting used to, since most folks probably haven't realized that going to the bathroom really winds up being a biological, biochemical, and scientific end process product. Your body produces daily a byproduct of metabolism, which needs to be recognized and assessed for what it is: A visual "guide" to your nutritional health status.

Medicine recognizes and gives credence to poop through many lab tests done on stool samples, which range from discerning if there are parasites, worms, infective/harmful organisms, e.g., E.coli, Yersinia, staphylococcus, shigella, salmonella, campylobacter, etc., blood, and even for pancreatic enzymes, which may foretell Pancreatic Elastase or Exocrine Pancreatic Insufficiency. So, humans, in my opinion, ought to have better respect for what poop is trying to tell us. In ancient Traditional Chinese Medicine, both poop and urine were examined for what clues they gave regarding a sick person's status, so evaluating poop is nothing new.

Before we try to read what a BM indicates, we first have to realize that since we usually eat three meals a day, each person should have a minimum of one healthy—not scrawny—bowel movement a day, preferably two or three, providing there is enough roughage and pure water in the diet. If that's not the case, I think you ought to consider constipation as an established and ongoing-condition.

I once had a client come to me and in going through the workup, I asked about daily BM habits. Every day—No! Every other day—No! Every third day—No! "So when?" I asked. "Every fifth day, but I'm not constipated," was the reply. I don't think so! Long story short, once that client got on to a proper nutrition program with daily fiber and fluids, etc., the poop began to flow like there was no tomorrow as, apparently, there was impaction or what's called sacculations[49] that began to release and empty out. That's how disease can get a foothold, causing inflammation, due to putrid or toxic matter being absorbed as "nutrition" through the intestinal tract wall, which then compromises the immune system and all body systems. You can't poison a body into wellness!

---

49 https://en.wikipedia.org/wiki/Haustrum_(anatomy) accessed 11-19-15

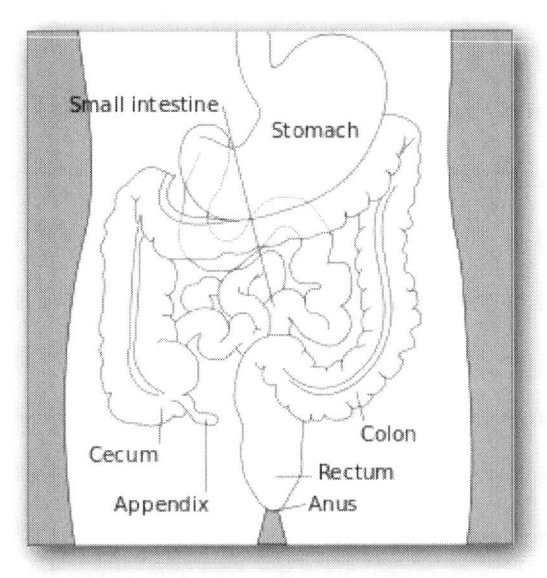

Graphic Source: https://en.wikipedia.org/wiki/Haustrum_(anatomy)
the Creative Commons Attribution-ShareAlike License

Perhaps, it would be beneficial for readers to study the *Wikipedia* site mentioned above to become familiar with digestion and elimination physiology in order to appreciate why we have to feed our bodies' cells properly in order to beat disease.

Getting back to the Bristol Stool Chart to learn more about what poop formations may mean, I truly believe that every type indicates the status of your gut's microbiome, or the microflora, that live in the intestinal tract, which do the Herculean job of processing foods, nutrients, and even manufacturing some of the B-complex vitamins.

Nonetheless, the human body truly is a magnificent 'machine' and deserves a lot of credit and respect for millions of tasks it does automatically and which we don't realize. Our bodies manufacture some vitamins like B-3 niacin, B-12 cobalamin—*if our gut is healthfully populated with lactobacilli, etc.*, vitamin D from sunshine, and vitamin K menaquinone, produced by the good bacteria in our gut. So, you see how important it is to have a proper ecological balance within the small and large intestines, which is where most of our immune system resides. Did you know that?

The type of a BM, according to the Bristol Stool Chart, indicates to my way of thinking at least, how our microbiome is colonized and functioning, and if it has the correct balance of microorganisms. In order to have that proper balance, food chemicals, sugar and synthetic sugars, fluoride, and refined starchy carbohydrates (white bread, chips, pretzels, popcorn, pasta, etc.) interfere with maintaining a correct, healthy gut microbiome population—even kill much of it, especially during an antibiotic regimen. Too much *Klebsiella Oxytoca* (a gut bacterium) in a stool sample also may indicate too many starches (including potatoes and brown rice) are being eaten. However, fiber from vegetables, in particular the complex starchy ones, is most essential for feeding the microbiome. Those starches, especially ones found in beans and legumes, are the preferred food of microbiome 'critters'. That being said, let's see what's going on with poop types.

Type 1 This type indicates to my knowledge of *natural nutrition* that the ecological balance of the microbiome is very much out of balance, plus the individual may be dehydrated or not drinking adequate amounts of clean, pure, non-fluoridated water on a daily basis. Constipation too!

Type 2 Indicates that there's too long of a transit time for chyme[50] in the intestinal tract, which probably is due to microbiome ecological imbalance. This type of poop can be difficult to pass and may tear intestinal wall tissue or make hemorrhoids bleed.

Type 3 Like types 1 and 2, indicates intestinal bacteria imbalance, plus constipation like the other two, but this type can be easier to pass.

---

50 https://en.wikipedia.org/wiki/Chyme accessed 11-19-15

Type 4 This type plops out very quickly with no straining, and is considered the perfect BM to have or strive for. Everything in the microbiome looks to be in balance!

Type 5 Is considered healthy too, but I question if some sacculations may be occurring.

Type 6 Can indicate a fast-acting colon, which may mean an overabundance of improper bacteria and low nutrient absorption. A high-quality probiotic regimen is suggested to bring it into balance.

Type 7 Diarrhea, which is not healthful and can lead to dehydration or masking other intestinal problems that should be addressed with your physician, especially if it lasts more than a couple of days. There could be food poisoning or bacterial (E.coli, etc.) contamination or other issues that need to be taken care of quickly. This is a definite indication of unhealthful microorganisms that need replacing with a high-quality probiotic regimen.

Additionally, I'd like to include another poop type: *mucus.* If your BM has a mucus coating, mucus threads, or there's mucus on toilet tissue, you need to bring that to a physician's attention, as you may have mucus- or ulcerative-colitis. IBD (Irritable bowel disease) is becoming more prevalent, especially since GMOs came on the food scene, or so it seems.

The last defining poop trait is *color*, which should not be overlooked, as it 'says' more than you might guess.

A normal healthy bowel is *brown* in color.

A *black* stool definitely is not normal, and usually indicates bleeding somewhere in the digestive tract. That abnormality must be brought to your doctor's attention immediately. However, certain things also can turn a stool black: blueberries and blackberries, black licorice, iron supplements, lead (Pb), and bismuth (OTC medication, e.g., Pepto-Bismol®).

Gray indicates serious digestive problems, or you are taking antacid medications, many of which contain aluminum hydroxide, which should be researched for what aluminum is capable of doing negatively in the body.

If the bowel or toilet bowl water has a tinge of *green*, which means that bile is present, you need to see a physician since there could be gall bladder or liver involvement.

Red indicates bleeding, usually from hemorrhoids, or a bleeding polyp. However, it can indicate bleeding in the lower intestine and should be investigated by a physician. Some variation of *red/maroon* usually appears after eating red beets. You also can expect to experience some reddish-pink urination too. That's normal for wonderful, liver-detoxifying, blood-building, red beets!

A *yellow or mustard-like* color indicates too much fat, which is not being digested, and you may need digestive enzymes. It also can indicate the presence of giardia (there are 6 types), a parasite usually found in unsafe water—drinking or swimming.

Now, here's the last definitive piece of information about poop: A healthy digestive and intestinal tract produces poop that has *NO odor!* I know you may find that hard to believe and accept. However, you will experience that once you balance your microbiome properly with a plant-based diet. Animal foods and red meat, in particular, tend to putrefy because they are difficult to digest properly and usually are eaten with improper food combinations. More plant-based foods, very little red meat, add a healthy probiotic supplement regimen, and your BMs positively won't have any odor. I think I can just about guarantee that. Odor indicates putrefaction in the intestinal tract or in the stomach, which usually manifests as bad breath or halitosis.

So, what are the "good bugs" that live in our intestinal tract?

There are numerous microorganisms that colonize the human gut, which some think of as the "second brain" in the body. As an example of what poop can tell about human biochemistry's end result regarding eating food—poop, fecal diagnostic testing can provide assays pertaining to pancreatic digestive enzymes, e.g., lipase, which breaks down fat, and chymotrypsin, which catalyzes protein. Long- and short-chain fatty acids results indicate just how efficiently fats are absorbed by the small intestine mucosa. Tests also produce the pH of fecal matter, plus if there is intestinal inflammation due to the "tell-tale" fecal lactoferrin being present.

What really gets the microbiome in trouble is the presence of unhealthful bacteria, parasites and their eggs, which poop also can provide. If parasites (there are numerous types) are present, you have to keep in mind that they eat and poop, too, and you, in turn, are absorbing their poop as nutrition. Yuck! So, now you can visualize what poop 'has to say' and why we ought to respect it for the wealth of information it can provide about our nutritional and health statuses.

The most efficient approach to seeding a healthy microbiome colony is to take a probiotic supplement that contains a comprehensive roster of *Lactobacilli,* e.g., acidophilus, casei, plantarum, rhamnosus, salivarius, brevis, bulgaricus, gasseri, lactis; *Bifidobacterium,* e.g., longum, bifidum, infantis, and *Streptococcus* thermophilus. If a probiotic doesn't have at least 13 to 15 types listed on the label, maybe you ought to consider looking for one that does.

The minimum daily probiotic supplement, in my opinion, ought to be 20 billion CFUs (colony forming units). However, for serious imbalances, up to 50 billion CFUs can be taken daily until gastrointestinal relief is acquired, and then maintain a 20 billion CFU daily regimen for all time. I think all probiotics should be refrigerated.

Another way to keep a healthy microbiome is to eat fermented foods such as sauerkraut, Kimchi, miso soup, Kombucha, tempeh (fermented organic soy beans), various fermented vegetables, and a sixteenth century fermented drink from Europe and Russia, *Kvass*.

There's something exceptional to remember about fermented foods. There's an abundance of microorganisms created during fermentation that produces vitamins, enzymes, antioxidants, beta-glucans, and phytonutrients—all extremely influential in beating diseases, especially beta-glucans, phytonutrients, and antioxidants for dealing with cancer.

I've given you a crash course or pep talk about poop, which I hope will impress upon you the importance of choosing and eating nutritious foods so that what your poop has to say about you will be most commendable.

Coincidentally, while writing this chapter I came across a *Thrive Market* article titled "What Your Farts Are Telling You About Your Health," which can be accessed online at http://www.care2.com/green-living/what-your-farts-are-telling-you-about-your-health.html.
I encourage you to read it, since not only is it humorously factual, you may gain additional insights into the importance of bowel health.

Something else that gut bacteria information is pointing to is whether type 2 diabetes is present in the body. Russian researchers have been able to link Blautia, Serratia[51] and Akkermansia bacteria. Even though

---

51 http://www.ncbi.nlm.nih.gov/pmc/articles/PMC4674628/accessed 2-17-16

those bacteria are found in healthy people, their numbers are greatly increased when type 2 diabetes is present.

Here are some of the highlights from that article:

- Sometimes passing gas isn't a laughing matter; it can be a symptom of underlying health problems! Did you ever think of farts that way?
- Flatulence is a byproduct of digestion that can be a symptom of food allergies, parasites, or gall bladder/liver problems, I offer.
- If you can clear the room after eating a bowl of ice cream, you probably are lactose intolerant and cannot digest lactase, the milk sugar found in cows' milk, cheese, and all dairy products.
- Pasta and gas go together if you are gluten intolerant, which can cause gas and bloating. Celiac disease could be at the root of all your gluten intolerances.
- Some medications can give you farts, or "toots" as the article calls them.
- A parasite—*Giardia lamblia*—also can cause *excessive* flatulence.
- And, lastly, passing some gas on occasion is normal for everyone.

However, when flatulence becomes chronic, putrid, excessively noisy, and even embarrassing, it's your digestive tract talking to you, I contend, trying to tell you to pay attention to every signal it's sending you: bloating, discomfort, odor, noise, and embarrassment.

Online Resources to Know About
How Your Gut Flora Influences Your Health
http://articles.mercola.com/sites/articles/archive/2012/06/27/probiotics-gut-health-impact.aspx

Mucosal biofilm communities in the human intestinal tract.
http://www.ncbi.nlm.nih.gov/pubmed/21807247

Biofilm: How This Slimy Coating Is Causing Chronic Fatigue, Fibromyalgia, Irritable Bowel, and More! http://bodyecology.com/articles/biofilm-how-this-slimy-coating-is-causing-chronic-fatigue-fibromyalgia-irritable-bowel-and-more

Biofilm Bacteria
http://thehealthyapple.com/biofilm/

Photographs of real biofilm
http://howirecovered.com/my-biofilm-exorcism/

Dr Michael Greger, MD, / NutritionFacts.org video on IBD/Crohn's disease, High Fiber Plant Food Diet
https://www.youtube.com/watch?feature=player_embedded&v=G-JuRjSrJPo#t=110

The types of microbiome species in the human gut: A short video explanation by Dr Michael Greger, MD. https://www.youtube.com/watch?feature=player_embedded&v=Zc_CncVcJK8#t=14

Here are some simple ways to boost the health and population of your microbiome:

- Eat a plant-based diet. That doesn't mean you have to give up meat entirely (unless, of course, you want to) but it should mean making plant-based foods the priority staples of your diet. That means including at least 7 servings of colorful vegetables, 2 or 3 pieces of fruit, a handful or two of raw nuts, some whole grains, beans, and seeds on a daily basis.

- Reduce your sugar consumption. Harmful bacteria and yeasts feed on sugar and can quickly throw off the balance of good to harmful microbes in your gut.
- Drink more [non-fluoridated] water. Water is needed to ensure regular bowel movements and bowel health. Sugared drinks and alcohol compromise the microbiome.
- Eat prebiotic-rich fermented foods daily. They include: Kimchi, sauerkraut, yogurt, to name a few.
- Eat plenty of high fiber foods like legumes (chickpeas, pinto beans, kidney beans, black beans, etc.), seeds (chia, flax, hemp, pumpkin, sesame, sunflower), and whole grains like brown rice, millet, amaranth, or quinoa (there are organic, sustainably-grown, fair trade brands available). Fiber keeps the bowels moving while preventing constipation and putrefaction from setting in.

Suggested Books

The Second Brain: A Groundbreaking New Understanding of Nervous Disorders of the Stomach and Intestine http://www.amazon.com/The-Second-Brain-Groundbreaking-Understanding/dp/00609

Heal Your Gut, Heal Your Brain
http://chriskresser.com/heal-your-gut-heal-your-brain/

Grain Brain: The Surprising Truth about Wheat, Carbs, and Sugar—Your Brain's Silent Killers
http://www.amazon.com/Grain-Brain-Surprising-Sugar-Your-Killers/dp/031623480X

Probiotics and Prebiotics: Do you know the difference?

Am I playing around with semantics? No! Probiotics and prebiotics actually are related nutritionally since both basically do the same thing, which is to provide nutritional sustenance for the gut and the microbiome flora colonies. But there is a technical difference between the terms.

Probiotics are defined as "live bacteria and yeast" that are exceptionally good for your gut and health, most often taken in supplement form, e.g., capsules kept refrigerated. The more numerous the strains—at least 15—in the probiotic, the better it is, I contend.

Prebiotics are foods, many eaten raw, which contain good bacteria that do the same as probiotics. Prebiotics include coconut water, kefir, Kimchi, Kombucha, miso, sauerkraut, tempeh, yogurt—foods that are digested in and by your gut to provide food for the flora that make up the microbiome. Prebiotics are found in plant fibers! Adults should eat between 25 and 40 grams of fiber a day! How much fiber do you eat every day? Other plant based prebiotic foods include raw garlic, raw onions, blanched asparagus, cooked onions, and brined pickles—not vinegar pickles, I suggest.

Most distilled white vinegars are very acidic (2.4 pH), which interferes with intestinal colonies, I offer. Distilled white vinegars most likely are made with GMO ingredients and from *grains*. Many folks can experience diarrhea or distress after eating vinegar. Why? One reason is gluten in the grains used to make the vinegar and, also, because vinegar can ream out the intestinal tract of microorganisms. There goes the neighborhood! Some folks believe in apple cider vinegar; I don't—its pH is 4.25 to 5.0, which is acidic. The lower a pH value, the more acidic something is. And when it comes to a damaged gut and microbiome, I believe in "soft and gentle" foods to bring peace to the gut's neighborhood. Fresh ginger as tea and an ingredient in recipes helps restore gastrointestinal integrity.

In the years that I was in practice as a consulting *natural* nutritionist, I can't tell you how many clients I saw who took to heart the apple cider vinegar folk remedy and only got worse. After taking their dietary history and realizing that fact, I recommended stopping ALL vinegars and seeding themselves with plain, full-fat dairy yogurt—4 ounces a day for 2 weeks first thing in the morning on an empty stomach—those were the days before probiotics could be purchased as supplements. I can't tell you how many folks thought I was a "miracle worker." It wasn't me; it was their microbiome responding to not being reamed out constantly. Personally, vinegar and black pepper are the two things I definitely avoid because of the damage they can do to the digestive tract for some folks, depending upon individual body chemistry.

One-size-nutrition does not apply to, nor fit, every person's individual biochemistry, I offer.

Here's something to think about: If you have taken antibiotics, you most likely don't have a healthy gut flora community. Do you experience: gastrointestinal problems; "leaky gut" syndrome; mucus colitis; Crohn's disease; inflammatory bowel disease; constipation; diarrhea; flatulence (farting); bloating or distended abdomen? If so, that's your intestinal tract talking to you using the only language it knows how to speak: discomfort when the microbiome neighborhood is not populated correctly.

Improper microbiome population can be one of the causes of inflammation and chronic diseases[52], something medicine has not quite wrapped its pharmaceutical arms around, I think. Probiotics and prebiotics are effective means to deal with and, hopefully, eliminate chronic inflammation using diet. Eat a diet built on plenty of fresh greens, colorful vegetables, and protein rich Omega-3 fatty acids. Chronic low-grade inflammation often is the precursor to atherosclerosis and clogged arteries.

One of the fallacies about keeping the gut happy is eating yogurt, either dairy or non-dairy, especially when taking an antibiotic. The term "antibiotic" means "against life" or "destroying life" which doesn't discriminate about what it kills in the gut, I offer. The good bacteria and flora become "collateral damage" in the antibiotic war on germs and microbes. Well, here's what I think you ought to know about yogurt if you really want to seed a healthy microbiome by eating yogurt.

First, no sugars should be in the yogurt; sugar *feeds* bad microorganisms! Neither should fruit be in dairy yogurt, as that's not a compatible food combination for proper digestive processes, which can cause more problems in the gut!

---

52 http://www.cell.com/cell-metabolism/abstract/S1550-4131%2814%2900311-8 accessed 2-16-16

Second, no chemicals, additives, preservatives, etc., as they can kill off fragile microbiome "critters" plus they add an acidic pH to the mixture, which only intensifies overall health problems, in my opinion.

On the pH scale, 7 is neutral while blood pH is between 7.35-7.45; Fiji water is 7.50; Evian water, 8.10; baking soda is 9—all alkaline. On the acid pH side, black coffee is 5.7; wine, 3; Pepsi, 2.53; Coca-Cola, 2.52; lemon juice, 2 with an alkaline ash though; stomach acid, 1.50-3.50.

It is my belief that maintaining proper pH values, while eating sufficient fiber quantity and quality from a predominately plant-based diet are the best and most effective ways to "eat to beat disease" and maintain optimum health, especially leading up to and in the latter years of life. Even though we all must die at the end of life, living should be about the quality of life and as disease-free as possible.

Sugar: Is it as sweet a treat as you think?

That rather rhetorical question probably will have you thinking more than once about how you feel about sugar, and all the edibles it goes into, after learning how processed sugars can contribute to disease development, especially weight, obesity problems, and act like fertilizer for cancer cells.

Before I get started giving you an abbreviated lowdown on sugar, I'd like to drop a thousand-pound clue: Sugar is what powers cancer cell growth. All cancers are 'fueled' by sugar[53] – or what turns into sugar in the body, i.e., starches, processed and junk foods, and simple carbohydrates.

For starters, let's talk about how much sugar the average person eats. According to some statistics, since 1983 sugar consumption has increased an average of 28 percent per person per year for a total of about 150 pounds a year per person! Shocking? Yes, especially when compared to 7 ½ pounds of sugar the average person consumed in the 1700s. Metabolically speaking, if you are overweight you need to be aware that, of the sugars you eat, your body stores 35 percent as FAT so that it can be converted into energy later. Furthermore, are you aware

---

53 http://beatcancer.org/2014/03/5-reasons-cancer-and-sugar-are-best-friends/?gclid=CL_JmYHrosk-CFYEfHwodhJsE1w accessed 11-20-15

that in the USA, 74 percent of food products contain caloric sweeteners or low-calorie sweeteners, or both?

Today's sources of refined, non-diet-type sugars are: cane sugar, beet sugar, corn sugar, and corn syrup. The last three most likely are from genetically modified crops, since those GMs are approved for use in U.S. food production and without having to be labeled as such on package ingredients and in advertising. Furthermore, 50 percent of the sugars in modern diets comes from high-fructose corn syrup (HFCS), found especially in fat-free salad dressings and soft drinks.

There are other natural plant-based sweeteners being touted as "substitutes" for sucrose (cane table sugar) and they are: agave nectar (cactus), honey (bees, which has been diluted with sugar water in China), stevia leaf extract[54] (aka *Truvia®*, *Pure Via®*), and sugar alcohols: mannitol (produced by the hydrogenation of fructose in starch or table sugar), sorbitol (obtained by a reduction of glucose usually from corn), and xylitol (extractions from either corn cobs or birch bark). Remember, anything made from corn in the USA probably is made from genetically modified (bt) corn. Several of the sugar alcohols are questionable, I think, since they can induce diarrhea, as can stevia leaf extract.

The list of artificial sweeteners includes: Acesulfame potassium aka *Sunett®*, *Sweet One®*; Aspartame, approved by the U.S. FDA in 1981, aka *Equal®*, *NutraSweet®*; Neotame aka *Newtame®*, approved in 2002 and can be used to replace molasses in cattle feed; Saccharin aka *Sweet'N Low®*; and Sucralose aka *Splenda®* approved in 1998. Artificial sweeteners travel parallel time lines, I contend, with the dramatic rise in obesity.

As of 2011-2012, a survey found in the USA, the following obesity rates: 35.8 percent of women aged 20+ were obese; 29.7 percent of that

---

54 http://regevelya.com/stevia-sweetener/ accessed 3-5-16

same age group of women were overweight; while 8 percent of that same age group of women were morbidly obese!

For U.S. men during the same timeframe and same age ranges, here are their results: 33.3 percent obese; 37.8 percent overweight; and 4.3 percent morbidly obese.

For children in the U.S. in that same timeframe, girls ages 6 to 11, 16.1 percent overweight; 19.1 percent obese; boys in the same age group, 16.8 percent overweight; 16.4 percent obese.

What do those percentages tell you? Have you lost a craving for sweets yet?

Ironically and rather late (April 2014) in the game of promoting artificial sweeteners, a study titled "Sweetened beverages, coffee and tea and depression risk among older US adults" stated that *"compared to nondrinkers, drinking coffee or tea without any sweetener was associated with a lower risk for depression, adding artificial sweeteners, but not sugar or honey, was associated with higher risks. Frequent consumption of sweetened beverages, especially diet drinks, may increase depression risk among older adults, whereas coffee consumption may lower the risk."* [55]

If you think *sugar-free products* are not impactful upon health matters, perhaps you ought to be aware of the 2015 study done by the Australian Oral Health CRC, which concluded *"sugar-free beverages, sugar-free confectionery and sports drinks demonstrated that many of these products contained multiple acids and had low pH values."* Furthermore, *"Researchers concluded that most of the products were potentially erosive, indicated by measurable softening and loss of tooth enamel following exposure to the products, and a reduction in healthy mineral levels in saliva."* [56]

---
55 http://www.ncbi.nlm.nih.gov/pubmed/24743309 accessed 12-3-15
56 http://www.oralhealthcrc.org.au/sites/default/files/Dental%20Erosion%20Briefing%20Paper_FI-

On page 10 of that report titled "BRIEFING PAPER: The potential of sugar-free beverages, sugar-free confectionery and sports drinks to cause dental erosion," it states that Coca Cola produced the *"highest amount of* [tooth] *surface loss."* The study's finding that really stuck out for me is, *"The most common cause of dental erosion is repeated exposure to acids in foods and drinks,"* something I like to point out and discuss: pH values and their impact upon health, especially from foods with vinegar, sugars, and chemical additives and preservatives, which produce acidic pH values. If acidic pH values can do that to the enamel surface of our teeth while chewing our food, what do acidic values do to digestive tract mucous membranes, the gut *microbiome*, and biochemistry in general? I heartily suggest reading that report cited in the footnote below.

For those individuals who experience gastrointestinal problems that just can't seem to be resolved or identified, perhaps the following information may be a clue as where to look for answers: Polyols—sugar alcohols used as low calorie sweeteners by food processors. Some polyols are monosaccharide-derived, i.e., erythritol, mannitol, sorbitol, and xylitol; whereas others are disaccharide-derived, e.g., isomalt, lactitol, and maltitol; plus polysaccharide –derived mixtures.

Interestingly, their raw material sources often are sawgrass oil, soybean oil, castor oil, rapeseed oil, palm oil, coconut oil, and some other oils—including animal. Are any of the polyols raw material sources genetically modified or subject to glyphosate or other chemicals, since the key polyol vendors are Bayer, Cargill, and Invista?

Sugar alcohols (polyols) are incompletely absorbed in the small intestine, which causes fermentation to occur in the intestines. Depending upon how much polyol one eats—either known or hidden in processed foods—there can be a laxative effect, abdominal gas, digestive discomfort,

---

NAL2015.pdf accessed 4-18-16

gut motility disorders, and those annoying stomach gurgling/rumbling noises, medically known as "*Borborygmus.*"

Furthermore, I have to warn you that there's an increasingly large variety of polyol-containing processed foods in supermarkets. Reading labels is one way possibly to know if polyols are an ingredient, since the FDA considers them as GRAS—generally recognized as safe! Sugar-free cough drops and candy, chewing gum, low-calorie soda and drinks often contain polyols.

Regarding the health-related issues usually associated with artificial sweeteners, I think what *Rodale's Organic Life* has to say makes a lot of nutritional sense.

> They trick your taste buds.
> They trick your gut.
> They mess with your hormones.
> They make you overeat.
> They increase the risk of diabetes.
> They're polluting your water.
> They're genetically modified.[57]

The part about tricking your gut is critical, I think, since artificial sweeteners can change the make-up of the gut microbiome that leads to unfavorable health consequences. Nothing points to that better than this article: "Artificial Sweeteners May Change Our Gut Bacteria in Dangerous Ways"[58], which talks about an Israeli study in which

> *10-week-old mice were fed a daily dose of aspartame, sucralose or saccharin. Another cluster of mice were given water laced with*

---

[57] http://www.rodalesorganiclife.com/food/trying-lose-weight-stay-away-artificial-sweeteners accessed 11-20-15

[58] http://www.scientificamerican.com/article/artificial-sweeteners-may-change-our-gut-bacteria-in-dangerous-ways/ accessed 11-20-15

one of two natural sugars, glucose or sucrose. After 11 weeks, the mice receiving sugar were doing fine, whereas the mice fed artificial sweeteners had abnormally high blood sugar (glucose) levels, an indication that their tissues were having difficulty absorbing glucose from the blood. Left unchecked, this "glucose intolerance" can lead to a host of health problems, including diabetes and a heightened risk of liver and heart disease. But it is reversible: after the mice were treated with broad-spectrum antibiotics to kill all their gut bacteria, the microbial population eventually returned to its original makeup and balance, as did blood glucose control.

However, in another study quoted in the above-mentioned article[59],

After consuming the U.S. Food and Drug Administration's maximum dose of saccharin over a period of five days, four of the seven subjects showed a reduced glucose response in addition to an abrupt change in their gut microbes. The three volunteers whose glucose tolerance did not dip showed no change in their gut microbes.

Glucose response refers to how efficiently sugar in the human body is metabolized. Frankly, I think everyone should know his/her fasting blood glucose levels. Taking a blood glucose test after fasting from food for 8 straight hours, normal blood glucose levels should be between 70 and 99 mg/dL. Normal blood sugar level readings taken two hours after eating (postprandial) should be less than 140 mg/dL.

If you do not know your blood glucose reading, don't you think it's about time you had that test taken? It's very important to know what your blood work is telling you and your healthcare practitioner about

---

59 http://www.scientificamerican.com/article/artificial-sweeteners-may-change-our-gut-bacteria-in-dangerous-ways/ accessed 11-20-15

your health. I heartily recommend that every person have an annual blood panel profile done every year starting at 30 years of age. Keep the results in a folder. Also, you can create an Xcel spreadsheet in your computer, and post yearly test results side by side, which becomes an excellent tracking tool, plus a way to see what needs attention, or if any red flags appear.

Sugar cravings, especially chocolate, are very hard to shake! I realize that and have seen many clients go through withdrawal and come out the other side truly grateful to have kicked the bad nutrition habit. I found that people who crave chocolate, more often than not, have some sort of blood sugar metabolism problem, i.e., hypoglycemia, or one that needs to be addressed, e.g., pre-diabetic.

However, like anything you want to gain control over, you have to "bite the bullet," as they say, and keep trying until you succeed.

One suggestion I can offer to overcome sugar cravings is to have grapes, raisins, raw unsalted almonds, pecans, or walnuts, trail mix without chocolate or sugar in it, on hand to pop in your mouth instead of candy, soda, an ice cream bar or cone, etc. The natural sugars in fruits (fructose and glucose, plus vitamins, minerals, and dietary fiber) will satisfy your body's cravings, plus provide nutrition too. After 7 days of not falling off the wagon regarding chocolate or other sugar and junk food cravings, you will find that you can—and will—beat the habit—no more "chocoholic"!

Here are some chocolate bar sugar contents in grams—are you aware of that?

3 Musketeers Bar 40; *Babe Ruth* 33; *Hershey's Milk Chocolate* 31; *York Peppermint Pattie* 25

Now, compare those candy sugar grams with fruit (grapes) grams:

One *cup* of red seedless grapes contains 23.37 grams of total sugars, plus vitamins, minerals, etc.

Let's see how nuts stack up. One hundred grams (3.5 oz.) of the following raw, unsalted nuts contain the amounts of sugar stated in grams, in addition to plant protein, healthful fats (Omega-3), vitamins, minerals, and fiber:

Almonds 4	Cashews 6	Macadamia 5	Peanuts 4
Pecans 4	Pine nuts 4	Pistachios 8	Walnuts 3

One almond weighs approximately 1 gram! Pecans, depending upon size, can weigh 2 to 15 grams.

Sugar-related Facts

Type 2 diabetes has increased threefold in the last three decades, since the 1980s.

Morbidity conditions acknowledged to be affected by sugar consumption include: acne, cancer, cardiovascular disease, depression, fatigue, hardening of the arteries, headaches, high blood pressure, hyperactivity, hypoglycemia, tooth decay, and violent behavior.

Where you don't expect hidden sugars: cereals, crackers, hot dog and hamburger buns, ketchup, mayonnaise, pasta sauce, peanut butter, salad dressing, soup, TV dinners, and most processed foods.

One 12-ounce can of Coke contains 10 teaspoons of sugar.
Sugar is an addictive substance, at least according to brain scans.
Sugar creates an acidic environment in the digestive tract.
Sugar suppresses the immune system and causes an overproduction of digestive enzymes.

Radioactive sugar in PET scans help diagnose cancer because cancer cells gobble up sugar. "*The radioactive sugar can help in locating a tumor, because cancer cells take up or absorb sugar more avidly than other tissues in the body.*"[60]

Sugar—like cigarettes—has had a great run, but relatively recently it's been recognized for what it does to affect health adversely. For anyone wanting to "eat to beat disease," it's absolutely imperative to remove all sources of sugar in the diet, except natural fruits. Candy, cakes, ice cream, pastries, etc. will never preoccupy you again, once you realize sugar's impact upon you and how well you feel after you've divorced yourself from its grip. However, there is something that I'd like to leave with you about sugar that I think is somewhat profound.

Rather recent research indicates that maple syrup may be able to fight inflammation. Quebecol, a molecule found in maple sugar—organically-produced, I hope, because formaldehyde sometimes is used in the filters attached to the trees during the tapping process—was identified by researchers at the Université Laval in Canada[61]-[62].

Now, here's something you may not realize, but is factual. There are numerous sugars[63] that can be included or even 'hidden' in processed foods. Do you know what they are? Why don't you try writing them down before you refer to the Resources below where I've listed them.

Another fact to keep in mind about sugar(s) is that high starchy carbohydrates turn into sugar during the digestive process. That's why folks who eat lots of starchy carbs wind up being overweight.

---

60 http://imaging.cancer.gov/patientsandproviders/cancerimaging/nuclearimaging accessed 3-5-16
61 http://www.sciencedirect.com/science/article/pii/S0960894X13009037 accessed 12-23-15
62 http://digitalcommons.chapman.edu/pharmacy_articles/73/?utm_source=digitalcommons.chapman.edu%2Fpharmacy_articles%2F73&utm_medium=PDF&utm_campaign=PDFCoverPages accessed 12-23-15
63 http://www.sugar.org/all-about-sugar/types-of-sugar/ accessed 3-5-16

> *If you are bitter at heart, sugar in the mouth will not help you.*
> A Yiddish Proverb

Resources

Neotame: Is This More-Dangerous-than-Aspartame Sweetener Hiding in Your Food?
http://articles.mercola.com/sites/articles/archive/2012/03/28/neotame-more-toxic-than-aspartame.aspx

Additional Information about High-Intensity Sweeteners Permitted for use in Food in the United States
http://www.fda.gov/Food/IngredientsPackagingLabeling/FoodAdditivesIngredients/ucm397725.htm#Neotame

Movie/documentary "Fed Up" An exposé about all the sugar in processed/packaged food
See the movie trailer at https://www.youtube.com/watch?feature=player_embedded&v=aCUbvOwwfWM#t=12

Added Sugar in the Diet
http://www.hsph.harvard.edu/nutritionsource/carbohydrates/added-sugar-in-the-diet/

Sugars that can be added, or even hidden, in processed foods
Corn sweetener, corn syrup, dextrose, fructose, fruit juice concentrate, glucose, high-fructose corn syrup, honey, invert sugar, lactose, maltose, malt syrup, molasses, and sucrose.

That, alone, ought to be reason enough to become an avid label reader while grocery shopping.

Do You Have a Sugar Addiction?

We've all heard of various addictions, but who would ever think that someone could be addicted to something like sugar, especially since it's in almost everything we eat? But, that's the problem!

Food processors use sugar in various forms: white sugar, fruit sugar, Bakers Special sugar, Confectioners or powdered sugar, Turbinado sugar, evaporated cane juice, brown sugar (light and dark), Muscovado or Barbados sugar, Demerara sugar, liquid sugars, invert sugars, plus the synthetic, man-made or low-cal sugar substitutes. Is it any wonder we have a "sweet tooth" or sugar addiction?

How do you know if you actually are addicted to sugar? One clue is that mostly everything you crave or eat has to taste sweet or be accompanied with a sweet drink like soda. Another clue is the type of snacks you usually eat: candy, chocolate bars, always popping "breath mints," or you are an admitted "chocoholic". What's your usual breakfast—sugar coated cereals, toaster pop tarts, donuts, pastries with cream and sugared coffee?

Another thing I think I'd like you to consider is the type of foods you crave. Some folks may not eat a lot of processed sugar containing foods and snacks, but "pig out" on a lot of fruit or starchy carbohydrates that turn into sugar in the bloodstream and affect blood sugar chemistry and levels.

Sugar addiction really exists and studies[64] have corroborated that. So, what can you do about kicking that addiction or, if you'd prefer, bad food habit? Well, like any biochemical addiction, one has to subscribe to detoxifying one's body. There are physiological clues that indicate sugar-dependencies.

Some are:

- Abdominal bloating or distention
- Acid reflux
- Belly fat or barrel-shape belly
- Brain fog / memory problems
- Diabetes or pre-diabetic [increased thirst, frequent urination, fatigue, blurred vision]
- Flatulence, gas (farts)
- Inflammation process in body picked up by blood tests, e.g., CRP / Westergren Sed Rate[65]
- Irritable bowel syndrome (IBS)
- Mucus: nasal, oral, or bowel
- Overweight or obesity
- 10 AM and 3 PM blood sugar "crashes"

In my opinion, there's only one way to detox and get the "sugar monkey" off your back, and that's going with what is called "cold turkey." If not, when you don't go cold turkey, you still are feeding that "monkey", which is counterproductive to beating it. Smokers find it hard to quit their smoking addiction, and no matter how hard they try,

---

64 http://www.ncbi.nlm.nih.gov/pmc/articles/PMC2235907/ accessed 1-20-16
65 https://labtestsonline.org/understanding/analytes/esr/tab/test/ accessed 1-21-16

if they don't or can't go cold turkey, in most cases, they keep trying and trying and trying to kick the smoking habit.

I contend that if you can go without sugar foods and starchy carbohydrates for five days straight, you are over that seemingly unsurmountable sugar addiction hump and you can—and will—kick the habit. I've seen it happen with many clients, but the first five days are hard to navigate, especially if you don't have the resolve to beat the sugar blues.

My suggestion is to carry little packets of raw, unsalted nuts, e.g., almonds, pecans, or walnuts, to munch on when you get a sugar/sweet craving. Always carry an apple in your briefcase so that just in case you really need to give in, you can cheat by eating an organic apple.

Soda addicts will have the hardest time of all, especially those who are addicted to cola type drinks.
Water, water, and more pure water is the secret, as it flushes the system clean. Plain hot tea or with lemon (green tea is an excellent antioxidant and "housecleaner") or coffee with some half and half can be helpful.

Going off sugar you will need to eat a little more fat in your diet to get you over the craving hump. You can find healthful fats in grass-fed butter; plain, not sugared or fruited, grass-fed kefir and yogurt; avocados; extra virgin olive oil on salads; raw seeds like pumpkin and sunflower (great snacks); unsalted, roasted peanuts or organic peanut butter (pure peanuts, no add-ins like dextrose, a sugar) eaten off the spoon.

Cheese can be problematic insofar as it can exacerbate gut microbiome, especially Candida Albicans, yeast infections that can play havoc in the stomach, intestinal tract, and female vagina, or jock itch in males.

Always keep in mind that you should not eat any foods to which you have allergies or intolerances such as gluten in grains; lactose in milk and dairy; histamine in foods (in fish it's called histadine); salicylates in processed or seasoned meats, wines, coffee and tea; and food processing chemicals, additives, and preservatives.

However, I can offer this ray of hope: The more you eat a healthful, balanced diet with plenty of complex carbohydrates from plant-based foods, the easier it will become to beat the sugar addiction. Fiber is a big helper in cleaning the body and equalizing body chemistry. Your diet will reinforce body chemistry to provide resources to fall back on, something it probably didn't have when you were eating what I'd call a "junk food diet."

The Effects of Food Processing on Nutrients

For those folks who aren't familiar with food processing procedures, I'd like to give a very brief overview of what happens to what's called "raw" product or farm-fresh foods after harvest.

If the raw product is grain, it most likely was "staged" in the fields for harvesting, which means that several days before harvest, the crop was sprayed with a glyphosate herbicide so that the entire crop had an even ripeness; the herbicide spray is used as a desiccant. Then, the harvested crop usually is stored in silos, which are fumigated to prevent vermin infestation. When grains, such as wheat, are taken to food processing plants, they are milled of their outer fiber covering where the precious water-soluble B-complex vitamins and fiber are found. The germ, where vitamin E-complex and fatty acids reside, is removed and what's left is called the endosperm, which is ground into starchy flours that are used to make end products or processed foods, i.e., cookies, breads, cakes, snacks, etc. However, the federal government requires that wheat flours be enriched with a few B vitamins and iron because, literally, hardly any nutrients are left in the flour!

For vegetables that are canned or become part of a canned or frozen product, they usually are washed with chemicals, pared, and cooked in high heat tubes, which can reduce fragile vitamin and mineral content due to evaporation or heat damage that, in some cases, can create free radicals, especially in foods with higher fat or cooking oil content, I contend.

That's why it is so nutritionally important to do what's called "scratch" cooking—to preserve and serve as maximum nutrient-dense food as you possibly can.

Now, to illustrate what's involved in denatured food, may I share with you the story of raw milk versus pasteurized processed milk, something that's been an ongoing "food war" for years regarding the nutritional value of raw "farm milk." The example I cite was published in the *Journal of Allergy and Clinical Immunology* (2016) DOI: 10.1016/j.jaci.2015.10.042 [66-67].

Researchers in Munich, Germany, verified that children who regularly drank farm milk as opposed to pasteurized store milk were less likely to develop asthma! Those children received immunological protection from the essential fatty acid Omega-3, which fresh, unprocessed milk contains.

Omega-3 fatty acids that remained in milk corresponded proportionately to the amount of processing farm milk went through, e.g., pasteurization, homogenization, and fat reduction. Furthermore, I learned that for calcium in milk to be absorbed, fat—butter fat in milk—must be present! What's happening to all those folks who drink low fat or skim milk and their bones? Can low fat or skim milk be a contributing factor to inflammatory processes[68] in the body like rheumatoid diseases, e.g., arthritis?

---

66 http://medicalxpress.com/news/2016-01-asthma-allergies-factor-farm.html accessed 1-27-16
67 http://www.jacionline.org/article/S0091-6749(15)01731-5/abstract accessed 1-27-16
68 http://www.drfranklipman.com/5-reasons-to-skip-the-skim-milk/ accessed 1-27-16

I'm not advocating the use of unpasteurized dairy products. However, I'm using raw milk versus processed milk to illustrate the fact that research is now documenting what natural food "faddists" have been stating for years: the beneficial and nutritional effects of raw farm milk and the denaturing effects of food processing.

Can Food Reduce or Eliminate Pain?

Ever since humans have been aware of their relationship to and with food, they have realized there are numerous benefits to be obtained besides eating, e.g., nutrients, fiber, satiety, and even medicinal qualities. Routinely, certain spices and plant-based herbs have been used prophylactically for centuries, if not millennia, in the treatment of pain, discomfort, and disease without debilitating side effects that often are produced by today's NSAIDS (nonsteroidal anti-inflammatory drugs)[69] painkillers.

In biblical times, olive oil and herbs were used medicinally. Some that were used include aloes, anise, bitter herbs, cassia oil, cinnamon and its oil[70], cumin, frankincense, garlic, hyssop, mint, mustard, myrrh, saffron, plus honey. We find that Manuka honey made by bees from Manuka (Tea tree) flower nectar in New Zealand is exceptionally higher in nutrients than locally-produced raw honeys.

Manuka honey is known for its natural antibiotic properties; it can help heal stomach and intestinal problems. It works extremely well in healing skin issues, especially acne and eczema. Manuka honey works well in pain relief for burn patients, decreasing

---

69 http://www.medicinenet.com/nonsteroidal_antiinflammatory_drugs/article.htm accessed 12-27-15
70 http://www.ncbi.nlm.nih.gov/pubmed/16710900 accessed 12-27-15

inflammatory responses. Manuka honey stimulates immune cells and works well for sore throats, allergies, and sinusitis. It can be used as a facial mask that fights free radical formation in the skin and for treating minor wounds and burns.

A tablespoon of raw Manuka honey a day spread on organic, whole grain bread or toast not only is a treat, but an effective way of getting a daily dose of this most therapeutic of naturally healing foods.

However, people with diabetic ulcers need to know that Manuka honey actually may interfere with their healing. The other cautions about Manuka honey use are: 1) it can raise blood sugar levels; 2) it can cause a possible interaction with certain cancer chemotherapy drugs; and 3) allergic reactions, especially in people who are allergic to bees.

Here are a few common foods that help in reducing pain and/or disease symptomologies:

Aloe Vera juice can help in acid reflux.[71]

Bromelain[72], an enzyme found in pineapples, works to reduce pain and inflammation of osteoarthritis and may help in IBD (irritable bowel disease).

Cayenne pepper[73] is a great anti-inflammatory response spice, one of the reasons I use it in cooking instead of black pepper. However, in sensitive people, it may induce stomach upsets. Cayenne pepper sprinkled generously on a cut, which won't clot or stop bleeding, works wonders within a few minutes.

---

71 https://www.youtube.com/watch?v=O890LxN6pSg&feature=player_detailpage#t=35 accessed 12-27-15
72 http://www.ncbi.nlm.nih.gov/pubmed/18160345 accessed 12-27-15
73 http://www.ncbi.nlm.nih.gov/pubmed/24235936 accessed 12-27-15

Chamomile tea is a no-caffeine herbal tea that is very relaxing and comforting, which can help ease the tension associated with pain.

Cherries, especially tart cherries[74] or their juice, work in relieving chronic inflammatory pain.

Flaxseed oil (high lignan), which contains an extraordinary favorable ratio of Omega-3 to Omega-6 fatty acids, has been used by cancer patients in dealing with breast[75] and prostate cancers.

Ginger is a great herbal remedy for stomach and digestive issues, in addition to being a pain reliever. It also works well for morning sickness during pregnancy. Fresh ginger relieves nausea and vomiting from motion sickness and cancer chemotherapy, plus it can reduce osteoarthritis pain. Gingerol in ginger helps reduce muscle pain and soreness, and has been known to alleviate menstrual cramps.

You will find that many of the recipes I share include fresh ginger.

Fresh ginger tea is easy to make and here's how: Peel and thinly slice 1 inch of fresh ginger and place into 2 cups of water; bring to a boil and turn down to simmer so it doesn't fizz/boil over. Simmer for at least 3 minutes. Remove from heat; add freshly squeezed lemon juice to taste and 1 to 2 teaspoons honey— Manuka from New Zealand has wonderful healing properties. Enjoy hot, warm, or iced.

Green Tea used on a daily basis can be very helpful in reducing free radicals, which cause inflammation and pain. This tea is recommended for all cancer patients.

---

74 http://www.ncbi.nlm.nih.gov/pubmed/15219719 accessed 12-27-15
75 http://www.ncbi.nlm.nih.gov/pubmed/25743093 accessed 2-21-16

Seaweed contains fucoidan, which reduces inflammation, plus all seaweed contains a lot more calcium than milk! Also, it's one of my favorite ingredients to add to a bowl of soup, or enjoy as a seaweed salad.

Turmeric/curcumin[76] can alleviate pain by interrupting or depleting a pain neurotransmitter, which then reduces the pain sensation. If you are taking blood thinners, definitely consult with your physician BEFORE taking turmeric/curcumin. It's been proven effective in cancer treatment and management.

Water not chemically treated is one of the most helpful and healthful fluids to stabilize body chemistry. Water is quickly processed in the body and can change body pH faster than most other foods, and yet a great percentage of people, especially teens, forego drinking water and choose soda or other liquids (coffee, tea, beer, etc.). Our bodies are 60 percent or more water; blood, 92 percent water; brain and muscles, 75 percent water; and bones about 22 percent water. It's thought that the lack of sufficient water intake by senior adults allows the brain to "shrink" thereby contributing to forgetfulness and dementia.[77]

Water is important for hydrating the inside and outside (bath or shower) of our bodies. Water, as designed by Nature, without other additives and chemicals, is what the body needs to keep healthy.

Soaking in a tub of warm water relieves muscle strains and also provides relaxing calm, especially if some Epsom salts or relaxing herbs like lavender[78] are added to the bath or soaking water.

---

76 http://articles.mercola.com/sites/articles/archive/2015/05/04/curcumin-turmeric-benefits.aspx accessed 12-27-15

77 http://www.waterbenefitshealth.com/water-and-brain.html accessed 1-28-16

78 http://umm.edu/health/medical/altmed/herb/lavender accessed 2-19-16

Organic Wine with no added sulfites can help relax the mind and spirit plus muscles, soothe achy joints, and ease pain too. Just don't overdo it. Red wine has ten times more flavonoids and more analgesics, which act similar to aspirin, than white wine.

What roles do food and nutrients play in our physical and emotional lives?

Quite a bit! For example, the mineral magnesium plays essential roles in 300 chemical reactions in the body, so if we are deficient in magnesium, we can experience all sorts of emotional and physical pains. A diet rich in leafy green vegetables, nuts, seeds, and legumes puts the body on the "auto pilot" control for pain-alleviating or pain-free living.

The human brain produces what are called natural "Feel Good Chemicals," which are: endorphins, oxytocin, serotonin, and dopamine. Other factors that also come into play that help those feel good chemicals include: exercise, humor and laughing, meditation, proper individualized diet, and the elimination of allergic-reaction foods from the diet.

Serotonin is a biochemical end product of complex carbohydrates in the diet, namely whole grains, brown rice, and oats/oatmeal. Avocado, Omega-3 fatty acid foods like salmon and nuts help relieve stress and inflammation. To assuage depression, eat foods high in folate (B-9) like asparagus and dark leafy greens. Other plant-based depression-fighting foods include: apple, avocado, beans, berries, mushrooms, onions, tomatoes, and walnuts.

Chia and sunflower seeds contain the amino acid L-tryptophan, which is a natural relaxer. Tryptophan is plentiful in almonds, bananas, cheese, chickpeas (garbanzo beans), dates, eggs, fish, peanuts, poultry, pumpkin seeds, red meats, sesame seeds, sunflower seeds, and spirulina (a supplement).

Endorphins are produced by the pituitary gland. Some of the recommended "feel good foods" to produce endorphins, I *wouldn't* recommend: chocolate, French bread, ice cream, and pasta. However, the plant-base foods that really up the endorphins include: bananas, ginseng, grapes, hot peppers, nuts, oranges, sesame seeds, and strawberries. However, the 10+ endorphin-producer is sex!

Which are the foods that will increase dopamine levels in the brain?

Almonds, apple, banana, blueberries, eggs, fish, ginseng, green tea, kale, oregano oil, peppermint, prunes, pumpkin seeds, red beets, sesame seeds, and strawberries help boost and balance dopamine levels.

Oxytocin is a hormone that helps reduce blood pressure and the bad feeling brain chemical, cortisol. It actually can increase pain thresholds, which means you can tolerate pain much better. It seems the mere ingestion of any type of food, increases oxytocin. However, I don't consider munchies and junk food as nutritious food. All the foods mentioned above are whole foods, not trademark concoctions!
Oxytocin actually reduces fear.

Foods high in saturated fats stress your body! Increase Omega fatty acids (3, 6) in your diet. Eat plenty of fiber, colorful vegetables, fruits, whole grains, and drink plenty of pure water. All that power-packed natural nutrition automatically will improve oxytocin levels in your brain and body.

Regarding the "Bad Feeling Chemical" – cortisol, other factors also come into play: fear, anger, tension, depression, poor diet and nutrition, food cravings, and the following foods, which can increase cortisol levels in the body: alcohol, caffeine, chocolate cake, cooking oils, fat-free and flavored/sugared yogurts, which can metabolize similarly as junk food in the body—I offer, low fiber carbohydrates, trans fats, plus food's glycemic index[79] ratings and the body's blood sugar levels.

Food Glycemic Index
The lower the food glycemic index score, as found in beans, fruits, nuts, and vegetables, the better the body's systems function, as they are biochemically balanced rather than spiking or dropping as with blood sugar levels that cause all types of weird sensations. A low glycemic index (GI) range is 0 to 55; medium range GI is 56 to 69; and the high GI range is 70 or greater. One of the vegetables with the highest GI is the potato, and how many folks live off fries and potato chips? Medium high GI vegetables include beets, corn, leeks, and sweet potatoes. All other veggies are low GI, with very low GI for most of the vegetables, especially leafy greens. Want to lose weight easily and deliciously, eat more veggies!

Foods that block inflammation in the body
Inflammation is at the root of all chronic diseases and premature ageing. However, the dietary choices you make can help block inflammation in the body just by what you put into your mouth. The following foods can help do that: Beets, berries, broccoli, cherries (tart), fermented foods, garlic, ginger, hemp oil, onions, peppers, pineapple, soy, spinach, turmeric, soaked walnuts that make them easier to digest, and whole grains.

---

[79] http://www.health.harvard.edu/healthy-eating/glycemic_index_and_glycemic_load_for_100_foods accessed 2-18-16

Two well-known and respected medical doctors in holistic/complementary medicine, Barry Sears and Andrew Weil, claim the anti-inflammatory diet is the best for maintaining overall good health. To that I would add one other thing: Remove all vinegar in any recipe or condiment in your diet!

What about protecting the brain from inflammation and memory loss?

Is there any food that can offer biochemical help? A study from the Salk Institute for Biological Studies that worked with mice indicates that a daily dose of the flavonol fisetin prevented memory loss and symptoms similar to Alzheimer's disease. Fisetin is a compound found in many fruits and vegetables, but is concentrated in two of my favorite foods, strawberries and cucumbers. Lucky me! Fisetin obviously protects brain neurons from the ageing process and those associated effects.

However, the lowly cucumber is more potent than you think. I used to recommend my menopausal clients eat a cucumber a day, including the seeds. They were amazed at how their hot flashes seemed to go away. Cucumbers provide antioxidants, e.g., vitamin C, beta-carotene, and manganese; anti-inflammatory lignans: lariciresinol, pinoresinol, and secoisolariciresinol; flavonoids: apigenin, luteolin quercetin, kaempferol; and triterpenes Cucurbitacins A, B, C, D and E. Who would have thought such a nondescript member of the melon family would contain so much nutrition? Here's what the cucumber's chemistry does in the human body. All the nutrients cited above, plus many more not mentioned here, inhibit the activity of pro-inflammatory enzymes, e.g., cyclo-oxygenase 2 (COX-2) and also by preventing nitric oxide overproduction that could increase excess inflammation.

Here's a great recipe for fresh, homemade cucumber pickles, which I love to eat. It's one that I learned from macrobiotic cooks.

Fresh Homemade Pickles
1 cucumber scrubbed well, or peeled if not organic, cut into thin slices
½ sweet onion, sliced into thin half-moon shapes
8 red radishes scrubbed well and cut into thin coins
½ tsp Himalaya pink salt
1 Tbsp. organic rice vinegar

Into a large mixing bowl, layer veggies starting with sliced cucumber, then sliced onions, ending with sliced radishes.
Sprinkle salt and vinegar over top.
Place a luncheon or salad plate on top of the veggies and then a heavy weight, something like a liter bottle of water.
Place the bowl on the side of the kitchen counter. The veggies will sweat and produce liquid, which you should drain off every hour or so. Keep the weight on top of the plate during the entire process, which should take about 4 to 5 hours. During the sweating and draining, the vinegar is leached out of the end product.
When there is hardly any liquid to be poured off, your fresh pickles are ready to be squeezed for a final release of liquid, fluffed using a fork, and placed in the refrigerator to eat as a side condiment, fresh salad, or topping for a tossed salad. These pickles will stay fresh refrigerated for 3 days, if you don't eat them before that.

Plant-based foods that can aggravate pain
Even though vegetables are extremely healthful, there's a classification—nightshades—that cause a lot of discomfort for folks with any form of arthritis, autoimmune disease, and gout. The nightshade vegetables include: eggplants, ground cherries, Goji berries, peppers of all types but

not black, potatoes, tomatoes, and tobacco, which you don't eat, but if you smoke it, you still get the nightshade effects in the body. Sweet potatoes and yams are not in the nightshade family.

There are several alkaloids in nightshades that cause discomfort. Solanine is in all nightshades, especially eggplants and potatoes. Tomatine is found in tomatoes and capsaicin in peppers. Those alkaloids inhibit the enzyme cholinesterase that regulates muscle flexibility. An alkaloid buildup can cause aches, inflammation, muscle spasms, pains, and stiffness.

I found that mushrooms often would start a gout flare up for some folks. Then there are food intolerances or allergies, which can play havoc with the body—anything from hives to diarrhea to palpitations and even sweating. Please refer to the chapter *Food Families and Allergies* for more information about foods you may not know could be part of your allergy profile and still eating.

High levels of inflammation can act similarly to high blood pressure, i.e., you may not even realize that you have it. The best way to check for inflammation is for your MD to prescribe one of several blood tests, e.g., C - reactive protein (CRP); Westergren sedimentation rate (erythrocyte sedimentation rate-ESR); and plasma viscosity detection (PV). It is *my personal opinion* that inflammation is at the core of high cholesterol levels too.

Can a nursing mom's diet affect her baby's colic?

Up to 40 percent of infants are affected by colic[80]. Dr Michael Greger, MD, discusses the need for paying more and efficient attention to colic

---

80 http://www.askdrsears.com/topics/health-concerns/fussy-baby/coping-with-colic/whats-colic-does-your-baby-have-colic-how-tell accessed 2-19-16

in infants in an online video[81]. What mom eats can affect the contents of her breast milk, which has gastrointestinal effects for her nursing baby. So what foods do a nursing mother eat that affect colic in her baby? They include dairy products, caffeine, gassy foods, grains, nuts, and spicy foods—more specifically corn, cow milk and products, eggs, soy, and wheat. Researchers found that dairy products (cows' milk, in particular) are the most offensive regarding colic, or so it seems. Keeping a food diary or chart cross-referenced with baby's colic episodes: time relative to feeding, intensity, and duration, are the best ways of getting a handle on relieving colic for that precious little bundle of joy and then, in turn, eliminating baby's reactionary foods from mom's diet.

Online there's a "Breast Milk Interactions Chart"[82] that every nursing mother ought to study to make certain she's providing the best "stress-free" breast milk for her baby, I offer.

Hopefully, after reading this chapter you can appreciate that what we put into our mouths really can exacerbate chronic pain; temper our thresholds for pain; and, even more importantly, how we can eat to relieve pain.

Resource to check out
Book: *Foods That Fight Pain: Revolutionary New Strategies for Maximum Pain Relief*
Author: Neal Barnard, MD
Publisher: Three Rivers Press

---

81 https://www.youtube.com/watch?feature=player_embedded&v=RTAAp4P0ln4#t=5 accessed 2-19-16
82 http://www.babycenter.com/0_breast-milk-interactions-chart_8788.bc accessed 2-19-16

Which Foods Help the Body Most in Managing Certain Diseases?

The human organism (body) has been evolving over eons of time utilizing three basic elements to survive and function: air, water, and food. We only can assume that prior to the Industrial Revolution (1760 to 1840), foods were not contaminated with chemical toxins manufactured by man. Naturally-occurring toxins such as found in poisonous mushrooms, ergot fungus, aflatoxins, and a host of bacteria were the primary poisoning agents found in food.

Ever since the end of World War II, when the pharmaceutical and chemical industries took off like greased lightning, hundreds of thousands of chemicals have come on the market. Food growers and processors can use any of 14,000 laboratory-made chemicals.

Many foods we eat daily, e.g., almonds, apples, cashew nuts, kidney beans, nutmeg, potatoes, rhubarb, and some stone fruits, contain certain toxins which we either don't eat—like the seeds or stones—or we have eaten them for so long—like potatoes (solanine) and tomatoes (atropine in the leaves and stems, which no one should eat or use for tea)—that we can tolerate them unless we have food allergies or certain diseases that "act up" after eating them, i.e., rheumatoid diseases react to nightshade family vegetables; similarly, people with gout can be bothered by mushrooms.

Below is a listing of some foods that are more efficient nutritionally to combat, protect, improve, or aid in healing of certain disease patterns. The legend I use is as follows:

BP for blood pressure
C   for cancer
Ch for cholesterol
D   for diabetes
H   for heart
I   for immune system
S   for stroke

Apples: H
Apricots: BP, C,
Artichokes: C, H
Avocados: BP, D, H, S
Bananas: BP, H
Beans: C, Ch
Beets: BP, C, H
Blueberries: C, H
Broccoli: BP, C
Cabbage: C,
Cantaloupe: BP, C, Ch, I
Carrots: C
Cauliflower: C, H
Cherries: C, H
Chestnuts: C, Ch, H
Chili peppers: C, I
Figs: BP, C, Ch, S
Fish: C, H, I

Flax seeds/oil as supplement: C, D, H, I
Garlic: BP, C, Ch,
Grapefruit: C, Ch, S
Grapes: C
Green tea: C, H, S
Lemons: BP, C, H
Limes: BP, C, H
Mangoes: C
Mushrooms: BP, C, Ch
Oats: C, Ch, D
Olive oil: C, D, H
Onions: C, Ch, H
Oranges: C, I
Peaches: C, S
Peanuts: C, Ch, H
Prunes: Ch
Rice, whole grain brown, wild: C, D, H, S
Not white/instant
Strawberries: C, H
Sweet potatoes: C
Tomatoes: C, Ch
Walnuts: C, Ch, H
Water, non-fluoridated: C
Watermelon: BP, Ch, S
Wheat bran: C, Ch, S
Yogurt: Ch, I

You will notice that the foods listed are what are referred to as *whole foods*—like those freshly harvested, rather than processed with chemical additives as packaged edibles. Whole foods are the keys to restoring and maintaining vibrant health. Plant-based or animal foods, which are not genetically modified nor engineered (GMO), offer the most nutrient values[83] when

---

83 http://www.organic.org/articles/showarticle/article-46 accessed 12-14-15

grown organically. With the exception of water, fish, and yogurt, all the above are *plant-based*, rather than animal foods.

Maintaining a higher percentage—around 75 percent—of your diet from plant-based whole foods is the *ideal recipe* for proper nutrition and health maintenance. However, for those individuals who need to have animal-based foods, I heartily suggest and encourage food sources that are produced from sustainable agriculture[84] and animal husbandry[85], free-range, and grass-fed[86], rather than animal foods produced by injecting or supplementing feed hormones and antibiotics, feeding GMO alfalfa, corn, and/or soy rather than grass for grazing animals.

Livestock raised by what's known as "factory farming", i.e., industrial agriculture[87], confines animals often to filth-ridden, box-like stalls or pens with no access to the outdoors, sunshine, and grasses under their feet, compounded by thousands of animals crowded together thereby negatively impacting animal mobility and health. Such conditions and pre-slaughter stresses allow stress hormones produced by animals raised for food products to lodge in their meat[88], at least in hogs[89] measured 24 hours post mortem.

Online there's a most informative website, "How Cattle Stress Affects Beef Tenderness and Flavor"[90], which I think everyone who eats meat ought to, at least, read and consider the difference between factory farmed and grass-fed meats.

---

84 http://www.ucsusa.org/food_and_agriculture/solutions/advance-sustainable-agriculture/sustainable-agriculture.html#.Vm7jOGzSn9I accessed 12-14-15
85 http://animalwelfareapproved.org/consumers/health-benefits/   accessed 12-14-15
86 http://www.sustainabletable.org/248/sustainable-livestock-husbandry   accessed 12-14-15
87 http://www.sustainabletable.org/859/industrial-livestock-production   accessed 12-14-15
88 www.steadyhealth.com/articles/hormones-in-animals-and-meat-quality accessed 3-6-16
89 http://www.sciencedirect.com/science/article/pii/S0309174004002736   accessed 3-6-16
90 http://www.grass-fed-solutions.com/cattle-stress.html   accessed 3-6-16

Factory farmed chickens also impact humans who eat them[91]. Free-range, pasture-raised hens produce higher quality eggs and meat. *Mother Earth News* did a study of pasture-raised eggs and chickens, and here's what they found:

> *"Our testing has found that, compared to official U.S. Department of Agriculture (USDA) nutrient data for commercial eggs, eggs from hens raised on pasture may contain:*
> - *1/3 less cholesterol* ▪ *1/4 less saturated fat* ▪ *2/3 more vitamin A* ▪ *2 times more omega-3 fatty acids* ▪ *3 times more vitamin E* ▪ *7 times more beta carotene."* [92]

For the record, I'd like to cite the nutrient content of large brown grade A eggs from grass fed hens as appeared on the inside box lid of Swiss Villa Eggs LLC. Cholesterol content is 185 mg or 62 percent of the recommended Daily Value. Sodium, 70 mg or 3 percent DV; saturated fat, 1.5 grams or 8 percent DV; protein, 6 grams representing 12 percent DV; 70 calories; 6 percent of DV vitamin A; 2 percent of calcium; and 4 percent of DV iron. At about 45 cents per one egg from grass fed hens, that's one heck of a nutritional bargain and bang for your food buck, I'd say.

---

91 http://www.motherearthnews.com/homesteading-and-livestock/raising-chickens/campylobacter-infection-zmaz10onzraw.aspx accessed 3-6-16

92 http://www.motherearthnews.com/homesteading-and-livestock/eggs-zl0z0703zswa.aspx accessed 3-6-16

Miscellaneous Diseases Affected by Diet and Nutrition

*I*n the Introduction to this book I stated that each topic I discussed could have a special book written about it. Furthermore, including comprehensive detailed information about the nutritional approach to numerous diseases would require this book to be close to a thousand pages. Since it's my desire to keep this book as interesting and brief as possible, but still try to turn you on to healthful eating patterns, I'm using this chapter to discuss briefly some diseases that occur frequently in today's modern lifestyles and which can be helped by lifestyle changes, the most important change being implementing a plant-based eating pattern on a daily basis.

Glaucoma

Glaucoma is a disease grouping, which damages the optic nerve that results in loss of vision and blindness. It can be prevented, and/or managed, by changing to a plant-based diet with plenty of leafy green vegetables and other nutrient-rich plant foods—something that's lacking in the sad American diet. Everyone over age 60 is at risk of developing glaucoma; for African Americans, over age 40.

My recommendation is that everyone starting at age 40 should have an eye exam along with a glaucoma test at least every two years and chart your eye scores every time. That way you can see how your chances of contracting glaucoma are stacking up test after test. I've had clients who, after maintaining a plant-based diet, had dramatic reduction in glaucoma test readings for both eyes—and readings stayed lower too!

Key nutrients in food that help glaucoma are the minerals zinc, selenium, and copper; antioxidants found in colorful vegetables; and vitamins A (beta carotene in vegetables), C (fruits, in particular), and E (whole grains, nuts, seeds, some leafy greens, avocado), plus a drastic reduction in caffeine intake from coffee, black tea, chocolate, and high-energy drinks, which usually contain some caffeine.

Specific plant-based foods, which nutritionally impact glaucoma, are those that are nitric oxide[93] boosting, e.g., leafy greens like arugula, celery, chervil, endive, fennel, leeks, lettuce, spinach, watercress; and the roots/tubers beets and celeriac.

Gallbladder – Disease and Stones

Hiding underneath your liver is a little sack called the gallbladder. Even though it's small, when it acts up, the pain is big time! Pain usually comes from gall stones that accumulate. They can be what are called "gravel" or stones as large as the size of small marbles. When those stones want to move out of the gall bladder and can't, you better get to a medical doctor or hospital emergency room.

However, it is my opinion that some gallbladder problems may result from food allergies that go unnoticed and unresolved, plus a diet rich in fatty foods, sugars, and starches. The best way to avoid

---

93 http://archopht.jamanetwork.com/article.aspx?articleid=2480455 accessed 3-8-16

gallbladder issues, which can include cancer of the gallbladder, is to get off the sad American diet merry-go-round and change to a plant-based, fiber-filled diet. Once you've had gallbladder removal surgery, digestive problems necessarily don't go away either! Some folks are bothered by acidic foods, fatty foods, and sugary foods. Cooking oils used to make chips and other greasy foods will take a toll too.

Since there is no gallbladder to act as a reservoir for the bile that the liver produces (400 to 800 mL a day)—the gall bladder's main purpose—fats and fatty foods often become problematic. Some folks find that they have to give up chocolate too.

Eating smaller meals post-gallbladder surgery can help.

Statistically, 42 million Americans suffer with gallstones and aren't aware that they have them! Each year one million people in the USA are diagnosed with gallstones, and there are half-a-million gallbladder surgeries a year! One of the sad after effects of gallbladder surgery is that some folks can experience IBS—irritable bowel syndrome. It's better to avoid all that by changing your diet now.

So, what do those stats tell you about the sad American diet based in greasy fast foods, fried donuts, chips, and sugary drinks?

Hypothyroidism
We are living in a time when there is a lot of radioactivity in the air from various sources including nuclear power plants and radioactive decay timelines from nuclear testing and atomic bomb detonations. Nuclear radiation, depending upon the isotopes involved, decay at varied half-lives from several minutes to thousands of years.

Unfortunate for humans, the human body is affected by radioactivity and the thyroid gland in the forefront of our neck, in particular. The end result of being exposed to all the ambient and freed radioactivity is an underactive thyroid, I contend.

For an underactive thyroid, which many people have today due to what I said above, plus Fukushima radioactivity that keeps encircling the globe from an uncontained core meltdown, plus women who have gone through menopause, often find their thyroid is sluggish. One telltale "body language" sign of a sluggish thyroid is that body temperature constantly can be below 98.6°F and in the 97 range.[94]

An underactive thyroid can make a person feel sluggish; feel cold; influence weight gain; experience depression, hair loss, constipation; have a hoarse voice; menstrual disorders, and interfere with fertility and reproduction, just to name a few symptoms caused by low thyroid function.

Older folks have a tendency to have a sluggish thyroid, which makes them feel cold, impacts memory, confusion, and dementia. Probably that's why they always wear sweaters, even during summer.

One of the dietary measures I take to keep my thyroid from becoming sluggish is to eat seaweed that's not from contaminated waters. Seaweed has plenty of natural iodine and trace minerals that most land-grown plant foods don't contain. Seaweed also is rich in selenium. The seaweeds that are rich sources of natural iodine are Kombu, Arama, and Hijiki. In the *Recipes from Catherine's Kitchen* chapter, there's a wonderful recipe for Hijiki Seaweed Salad.

Other dietary and nutritional fortification for the thyroid include eating plenty of herbs like fresh cilantro, cinnamon, ginger, and

---

94 http://www.regenerativenutrition.com/content.asp?id=574 accessed 3-8-16

turmeric, as they can boost metabolism in people with underactive thyroids. Seaweed also is a help-mate for losing weight.

The other food issue surrounding hypothyroidism is limiting foods that are "Goitrogens" such as cruciferous vegetables: Bok choy, broccoli, cabbage, cauliflower; papaya, radish, and soy products. Goitrogens are compounds in some foods that interfere with thyroid function, i.e., they disrupt thyroid hormone production by interfering with iodine uptake by the thyroid gland.

Foods that can boost thyroid function include: animal proteins (meat, dairy, eggs) from pasture-raised animals without GMO feed and hormones; proteins in seeds and nuts; colorful vegetables; and non-gluten grains, e.g., amaranth, buckwheat, brown rice, cornmeal, oats, and quinoa.

Probiotics (discussed in another chapter) are important for individuals with low thyroid activity because, if the gut microbiome is not in balance, thyroid activity can fluctuate.

Immune System

The immune system's workhorse is the intestinal tract, where most of the human immune system resides. Did you know that? Well, that simple factoid ought to inspire you to pay more attention to what you feed your body and, particularly, how it's processed into nutrition once it gets out of the stomach and travels its way through 32 feet of intestines.

One of the unsuspected interferences with proper nutrition and health is a condition called "Small Intestinal Bowel Overgrowth" or SIBO. SIBO encompasses many of the problems of leaky gut and Irritable Bowel Syndrome (IBS), plus malabsorption of vitamin B12.

The altered overgrowth of gut bacteria (SIBO) has numerous causes: antibiotics; prescription drugs, e.g., prednisone and proton-pump inhibitors; poor bowel motility; insufficient digestive enzymes; and chronic pancreatitis.

Starchy foods are to be avoided, as are grains containing gluten. Other foods to avoid are: alcohol, caffeine, coffee, and fried foods. Remember, caffeine is in chocolate as theobromine[95]. Prebiotics and probiotics are a must for dealing with SIBO. See the chapter that deals with them.

For individuals who can't seem to find relief, maybe you ought to talk with your healthcare professional about taking a Stool Culture test for bacteriology, microbiology, and yeast. That will find the bad "bugs" that need to be dealt with, and which may require specific pharmacology and targeted nutritional advice.

Additionally, you may have to consider what's called the Low FODMAP Diet. FODMAP is the acronym for Fermentable Oligo-Di-Monosaccharides and Polyols, which are certain sugar carbohydrates found in specific foods. Stanford Hospital & Clinics has an online FODMAP diet[96].

Obesity and Weight Loss

Since obesity is a compounding health problem in most diseases[97], I would imagine that anyone who is twenty pounds overweight ought to be dedicated to finding a diet he or she can stick with as a way of life to

---

95 https://en.wikipedia.org/wiki/Theobromine accessed 3-8-16
96 https://stanfordhealthcare.org/content/dam/SHC/for-patients-component/programs-services/clinical-nutrition-services/docs/pdf-lowfodmapdiet.pdf accessed 3-8-16
97 http://www.ncbi.nlm.nih.gov/books/NBK44210/ accessed 3-8-16

keep off the pounds, especially as they grow into old age. Children need to learn at an early age how to eat nutritiously[98].

The key to automatic weight loss and maintenance, in my opinion, is a plant-based diet that forsakes all the desserts no matter that they are made from plant foods. For a sweet tooth, satisfy it with fresh whole fruit. A plant-based diet provides roughage that is nutritious and filling, plus offers a lot less calories than menus built around fast food restaurants, snack foods, diet sodas and drinks.

Furthermore, capsaicin in hot peppers, chili powder, garlic, ginger, and green tea are foods that can increase your body's metabolism; they are called "thermogenic" foods, meaning foods that require more energy to burn and, thus, boost metabolism. That's known as the "*Thermogenic Effect of Foods*," and you can learn more about that at eMed Expert online at http://www.emedexpert.com/tips/metabolism-tips.shtml#ref1.

Pure water also has the ability to boost the rate at which your body burns calories, according to the German scientific study "Water-induced Thermogenesis" published in *The Journal of Clinical Endocrinology and Metabolism*, 2003 Dec; 88 (12):6015-9.

I had nutrition clients who could not believe how much weight they lost while eating as much plant foods as they did all while keeping their blood sugar balanced; were not hungry; and felt better than they had since their teenage years.

My contention is that once you can make up your mind to stick with a plant-based diet, even though you may eat grass-raised, GMO-free animal products a few times a week, you will lose weight. You can eat so much more nutritious food in comparison to high calorie starchy

---

[98] http://bgr.com/2015/10/14/american-obesity-school-lunches/ accessed 3-8-16

carbohydrates, sugary drinks, beer, snack foods out of packages, fancy and expensive lattés, and fast food restaurant menus.

There's a book published in January of 2016, *Always Hungry? Conquer Cravings, Retrain Your Fat Cells & Lose Weight Permanently* by David Ludwig, MD, PhD, which may help you to conquer any weight problems.

What's the Story about Toxic Sprays Used on Crops?

The Environmental Working Group (EWG) has done a fantastic job of letting consumers know the real deal stories about pesticides and herbicides sprayed on crops growing in the fields[99].

EWG's annual "Dirty Dozen Shopper's Guide to Pesticides in Produce" (2015 version) includes apples, celery, cherry tomatoes, cucumbers, grapes, nectarines, peaches, potatoes, snap peas, spinach, strawberries, sweet bell peppers, hot peppers, and kale/collard greens as being the most heavily sprayed crops.

If you have no choice but to buy any of the "Dirty Dozen," then wash or do a quick-soak in a "Fruit and Vegetable Wash" that does NOT contain chemicals, but is made from plant oils and citrus seed extracts. You also can apply the wash directly to an apple or eggplant; massage it around for at least 30 seconds; and then rinse thoroughly.

EWG's "Clean Fifteen Shopper's Guide to Pesticides in Produce" states that asparagus, avocadoes, cabbage, cantaloupe, cauliflower,

---

99 http://www.ewg.org/foodnews/summary.php accessed 1-8-2016

eggplant, grapefruit, kiwi, mangoes, onions, papayas, pineapples, sweet corn, sweet peas, and sweet potatoes are the least sprayed crops with relatively few pesticide concentrations detected. However, if any of those are genetically-modified, then they are routinely doused with glyphosate[100].

Without proper labeling of genetically-modified foods/crops, one really does not have any indication as to how food is grown with the exception of the "organically-grown" label and certification. Granted, with all the chemtrail spraying overhead, the only assurance we have with the organic label and certifications is that toxic chemical sprays and fertilizers were not used in their growing cycles.

The prefix number 9—usually larger than the four following numbers—indicates organically grown.

According to Green America's website[101], here's what's genetically modified:

Soy GM since 1996 affecting 94 percent of the USA soy crop [soy oil]

Cottonseed GM since 1996 affecting 90 percent of the USA cotton crop [cottonseed oil]

Corn GM since 1996 affecting 88 percent of the USA corn crop [corn oil]

Canola oil GM since 1996 affecting 90 percent of the USA canola crop [cooking oil]

U.S. papaya GM since 1998 affecting 80 percent of the USA papaya crop

Alfalfa GM since 2005 and used as cattle feed, which can taint meat and animal products

---

100 http://www.ewg.org/foodnews/?gclid=CMOsmrPImsoCFdCPHwod1DIL7Q accessed 1-8-2016
101 http://action.greenamerica.org/p/salsa/web/common/public/signup?signup_page_KEY=7608&tag=adwords&gclid=CO7LlL7LmsoCFVMWHwodFWMORw accessed 1-8-2016

Sugar beets GM since 2005 affecting 95 percent of the USA sugar beet crop

Milk GM since 1994 by the recombinant bovine growth hormone (rBGH) being injected into 17 percent of USA cows

Aspartame GM since 1965 is derived from GM microorganisms and is used in over 6,000 products, especially low calorie edibles.

How do shoppers know what's GMO and what's not, since there is no GMO labeling required in the USA? The Institute for Responsible Technology publishes online their "Non-GMO Shopping Guide," which you can find at http://www.nongmoshoppingguide.com/. Just click on the food photographs for detailed listings of non-GMO foods and brands.

I cannot impress upon you how important health-wise it is not to eat GMO-produced foods or eat grains that have been sprayed with glyphosate pre-harvest. Gastrointestinal and digestive problems have increased. *"The percentage of Americans with three or more chronic illnesses jumped from 7% to 13% in just 9 years; food allergies skyrocketed, and disorders such as autism, reproductive disorders, digestive problems, and others are on the rise."*[102]

One guaranteed way of not purchasing and unwittingly eating heavily-herbicided food is to purchase organically-grown fresh and processed foods. Amy's is a trusted brand name canned and frozen foods producer. Farmers markets provide local, fresh food, but you need to ask the farmer about the produce you are purchasing; if it's been sprayed, and with what.

There are many food producers and processors with national brand names that you can count on being safe; they are listed in the IRT's shopping guide.

---

102 http://responsibletechnology.org/10-reasons-to-avoid-gmos/ accessed 1-8-2016

Even though, theoretically as of the time I'm writing this book, there supposedly is no GM-wheat being grown or sold in the USA[103], there is, though, a harvesting trick farmers employ whereby three or four days before harvesting grain and legume crops, they go through a staging procedure of spraying crops to effectuate an even ripeness, which the herbicide glyphosate apparently accomplishes. Glyphosate has been found as residues in harvested crops[104]-[105].

---

103 http://beyondpesticides.org/dailynewsblog/2015/01/monsanto-once-again-developing-herbicide-resistant-wheat/ accessed 1-8-2016
104 http://www.sciencedirect.com/science/article/pii/S0308814613019201 accessed 1-8-2016
105 http://healthimpactnews.com/2014/alert-certified-organic-food-grown-in-u-s-found-contaminated-with-glyphosate-herbicide/ accessed 1-8-2016

Is There Such a Disorder as "Toxic Body Syndrome"?

What is toxic body syndrome, you may be asking. It's *my hypothesis,* and the possible explanation, as to why there are so many chronic forms of disease, not only in older persons, but in the very young and at extremely high occurrence rates.

Statistically, we saw that in 1960 only 1.8 percent of children experienced illnesses that lasted more than three months. However, by 2004 that rate had risen to 7 percent of U.S. children having chronic-type symptoms. The chronic conditions that were the top three in the USA in the 1970s were obesity, asthma, and attention deficit hyperactivity. Chronic conditions now affect between 15 and 18 percent of children and teens[106].

What about adults? Here's what the U.S. CDC cites as statistics for chronic disease in adults:

---

106 http://abcnews.go.com/Health/Healthday/story?id=4507708&page=1 accessed 2/1/16

As of 2012, about half of all adults—117 million people—had one or more chronic health conditions. One of four adults had two or more chronic health conditions.[107]

So, what does the CDC classify as chronic diseases? Heart disease, stroke, cancer, diabetes, obesity, and arthritis, which CDC says are among the most costly and *"preventable of all health problems."*

Yes! They certainly can be prevented. However, the two best means of preventing them are a nutritious diet plus a lifestyle avoiding toxic chemicals in food, water, and scented products that inundate the market and for which consumers wind up being apparent "pushovers."

In 2009, I wrote the book, *Our Chemical Lives And The Hijacking Of Our DNA, A Probe Into What's Probably Making Us Sick,* which discussed in great detail (over 400 pages) what you need to know about toxins affecting your health. That book is available on Amazon.com, and may be helpful to you in understanding why I'm writing this chapter.

Remember, I'm a retired consulting *natural* nutritionist who, in my practice, saw thousands of clients who, I'd say, experienced "toxic body syndrome." One woman, in particular, came to me with such memory problems that she was super-frustrated. After working with me (detox program and educating her about eating nutritiously and lifestyle changes), she was able to file a joint federal income tax return for her husband and herself! A few years ago, she found my email address online and sent me an email from Florida, where they retired, to say how much she appreciated what I taught her; she still practices her nutrition "religiously"; and that she's enjoying very good health in her 80s!

---

107 http://www.cdc.gov/chronicdisease/overview/ accessed 2/1/16

That story is only one of hundreds I can share, including those clients who were on disability, but once they got detoxed and rebuilt their bodies using healthful, natural nutrition practices, went off disability and returned to work. Or children who were impaired due to high lead in their bodies.

Detoxified of the lead, they went from failing in their school grades to being honor roll students.

The problem that everyone – and mostly medical doctors – doesn't want to accept is that man-made chemicals are poisons—in any amount, too. Any amount in the human body interferes with biochemistry, DNA/RNA sequencing—gene expression, and causes adverse health effects, especially resulting from the cumulative effects of all the toxic chemicals humans are forced to eat, drink, breathe, and be exposed to minute-by-minute – 24/7/365, plus vaccine chemicals[108] injected during vaccinations.

What are those ubiquitous chemical exposures?

Frankly, they are too numerous to recite, but here are just a few of the more egregious: Chemtrails sprayed from airplanes into skies overhead that fall to the ground and we are forced to breathe aluminum particulates, strontium, barium, viruses, and other 'goodies' in that Solar Radiation Management / weather geoengineering mix; fluoride in municipal water systems since the 1950s, in toothpastes and at the dentist's office; toxic food processing chemicals ever since shortly after the end of World War II; pesticide and herbicide sprays in agriculture and food production; veterinary pharmaceuticals and hormones for animal husbandry, meat and milk production, and the egg industry; toxic household cleaning products; synthetic wood products and cabinetry with toxic formaldehyde gas out; scented

---

108 http://www.cdc.gov/vaccines/pubs/pinkbook/downloads/appendices/B/excipient-table-2.pdf accessed 3-5-16

products like candles and room 'fresheners'; genetically modified 'phoods' with foreign DNA inserted, which are modified to tolerate the inordinate amounts of the herbicide glyphosate that are sprayed on GMO crops, and the list goes on and on.

We breathe in toxic fumes that cause health problems for our bronchi, lungs, and liver—the brain gets foggy too. We eat and drink toxic chemicals, which are offered as colorings, flavors, additives, preservatives, etc., and yet we really don't know the combined synergistic effects of innumerable chemicals interacting constantly within human body biochemistry every day of our lives. My contention is that the result is "toxic body syndrome." Does that make any sense?

How can anyone with scientific/medical knowledge not say that all those countless chemicals do not overload biological functions, pathways, and enzyme systems? By the way, even the FDA doesn't know all the chemicals in our food[109]-[110]!

However, I do believe if the medical professions were to come down hard on chemicals that action would catapult the pharmaceutical industry into a tizzy and probably put some out of business. Why? Because pharmaceuticals are pure man-made toxic chemicals sold under legal licensure called prescription drugs. And, nothing is as contaminated with toxins as vaccines, which everyone is mandated and subjected to receive from birth to old age. It is my unvarnished opinion from years of researching vaccine literature that vaccines are a primary factor in the cause of the rise in chronic childhood diseases. Combine that with poor diet and nutrition, so what do you have? A captive—and literally growing—sick clientele who

---

109 http://ecowatch.com/2014/04/12/fda-food-nervous/ accessed 2-1-16
110 http://www.fda.gov/Food/IngredientsPackagingLabeling/FoodAdditivesIngredients/ucm115326.htm accessed 2-1-16

will 'need' and receive more toxic chemical intervention in the way of prescription drugs, possibly mood enhancing ones like SSRIs. What is chemotherapy except toxic drugs designed to kill cancer cells? Why do patients lose their hair and experience the horrors of cancer treatments, e.g., "chemo brain," if those drugs are not poisonous? And some of the drugs given to cure cancer actually can cause cancers in the future[111].

All those toxins take their toll on the body's organs and systems. If those toxins can be released from the body, which most can't unless detoxified with specific protocols to go after them, the body gets sicker and sicker[112]. That's why I believe that eating a nutritiously clean and healthful diet is a critical key to regaining, managing, and maintaining vibrant health.

Many of the foods recommended in this book [broccoli—especially sprouts, citrus: lemons, oranges, limes, fruits, garlic, green tea, leafy greens, mung beans, nuts (raw), Omega 3-fatty acids, seeds, vegetables (raw and cooked *a la dente*)] have automatic detoxifying properties built in, which will help your body to detoxify using a "slow motion" routine, and with every bite you eat.

However, regarding detoxification if you are so inclined, I recommend a supervised detox protocol/program, which many holistic physicians offer and supervise. That, coupled with eating as suggested in this book, ought to convince you that "eat to beat disease" truly is within your grasp and extremely rewarding.

Toxic body syndrome, in my opinion, leads to some of the recognized "modern diseases" such as Multiple Chemical Sensitivity

---

111 http://www.cancer.org/cancer/cancercauses/othercarcinogens/medicaltreatments/secondcancerscausedbycancertreatment/second-cancers-caused-by-cancer-treatment-chemotherapy accessed 2-2-16

112 http://www.naturesintentionsnaturopathy.com/body-detox/signs-and-symptoms-of-a-toxic-body.htm accessed 2-1-16

(MCS)[113] aka "environmental illness" or "sick building syndrome," and what's called "Electromagnetic hypersensitivity" (EHS) when a person is compromised in numerous ways from microwaves emitted by cell phones and towers, utility company AMI smart meters, Wi-Fi, routers, monitoring devices and many of the "smart" gadgets and appliances, which can send and receive information, data, or voice.

The American Academy of Environmental Medicine publishes a three-page list of medical conditions at https://aaemonline.org/pdf/AAEMEMFmedicalconditions.pdf that are exacerbated by EMFs. Become acquainted with symptoms that can result from electromagnetic radiofrequencies, microwaves, Wi-Fi, smart meters, and smart appliances.

If you've never heard of EHS, the World Health Organization (WHO) recognizes it and MCS as legitimate health problems. In a May 31, 2011 Press Release, WHO stated, *"The WHO/International Agency for Research on Cancer (IARC) has classified radiofrequency electromagnetic fields as possibly carcinogenic to humans (Group 2B), based on an increased risk for glioma, a malignant type of brain cancer, associated with wireless phone use."*

A team of researchers identified a blood test that can identify both EHS and MCS in a person.[114-115]

Toxicity can come from many sources, including OTC and prescription drugs/medications. When the body is saturated with toxins it can no longer function in a state of wellness and disease sets in. One prime example of that can be found in various industries where workers have

---

113 http://www.webmd.com/allergies/multiple-chemical-sensitivity accessed 2-2-16
114 http://www.hindawi.com/journals/mi/2014/924184/ accessed 2-2-16
115 http://www.activistpost.com/2015/11/electromagnetic-hypersensitivity-from-microwave-technology-finally-medically-proven.html accessed 2-2-16

been exposed to toxic metals or chemicals, e.g., asbestos. Certainly, everyone is familiar with what lead (Pb), asbestos, and DDT can do in the body. That's why there is the federal government U.S. Department of Labor's Occupational Safety and Health Administration (OSHA)[116], an agency whose main concern is to inform workers about health hazards in the workplace.

In today's fast moving world of science and technology, it is incumbent upon everyone to learn how to protect themselves, plus ask questions about what you perceive to be affecting your health and/or wellbeing. You have the right to be well and not made sick by anyone or anything, I contend.

I'd like to quote Mike Adams because I think what he says fits in with my contention of toxic body syndrome:

> *"The deceptions are quite incredible. One company that imports nearly 100 percent of the rice protein used by all the vegan protein manufacturers in the United States is fully aware that their product contains high concentrations of toxic lead, cadmium, tungsten, and mercury. On their website, however, they claim their material is "Prop 65 compliant," referring to Proposition 65 in California."*[117]

To that, add this from Adams' book, *Food Forensics,* which further points to toxic body syndrome:

> *"In September 2013, the CDC issued its updated fourth National Report on Human Exposure to Environmental Chemicals, detailing more than 201 chemical substances that have been identified in blood serum and urine levels throughout the U.S. population.7*

---

116 https://www.osha.gov/html/a-z-index.html   accessed 2-2-16
117 Mike Adams, Food Forensics, (Dallas, TX: BenBellaBooks, 2016), Pg. 5.

These can be ingested, absorbed, stored, excreted, metabolized, or bound to other compounds—potentially interacting with, blocking, or amplifying reactions within the body." [118]

As I've said many more times than I can count, "You can't poison a body into wellness."

---

[118] Ibid. Pg. 14. 7 http://www.cdc.gov/exposurereport/pdf/FourthReport_UpdatedTables_Sep2013.pdf#page=1&zoom=auto,0,800

What Role Does Diet Play Regarding Cancer?

More and more attention is being directed toward the role of food and chemicals in contracting cancer. Food processing chemicals have been highlighted as probable factors for quite some time. Red meat and dairy products get "thumbs down." Everyone probably is familiar with the role that cruciferous (Cole or cabbage family) vegetables play in preventing, treating, and managing cancer. But what exactly is in some foods more than others that predisposes or causes cancers to form?

First and foremost, other than toxic poisons/chemicals, is the lack of nutrients that can be due to various factors starting with seeds, chemical soil enhancements, herbicides, food storage and processing, the manner of food preparation/cooking, and individual food choices. If there are very little nutrients in food, especially synthetic and/or processed foods, the body receives no nutritional resources to maintain life functions at cellular levels.

Personally, I think if people knew and understood the role of certain compounds in foods that program abnormal cell growth, they would be more amenable to changing their diets and eating much more in the way of plant-based, unprocessed, whole, and raw foods.

Cows' milk, in particular, stimulates TOR (Target of Rapamycin) proteins, which is referred to as the "engine-of-ageing-enzyme" that, basically, regulates growth and life span, plus plays a role in brain development, learning, and memory. The biochemical factors in cows' milk now are being regarded as "species specific endocrine signaling systems" that, in turn, hyper-activate TOR and promote cell growth and proliferation, including rogue cancer cells. That's the reasoning for eliminating dairy, especially in cancer patients, I feel.

There's a balance that has to be maintained between protein synthesis and protein degradation, which TOR proteins regulate. The signaling occurs when there are sufficient nutrients for protein synthesis.

So, how can we effectively modulate TOR signaling? There are two ways: one is a very low calorie intake, which I don't advise, and the other is by reducing animal protein intake, especially cows' milk products and other animal proteins, while increasing daily dietary intake of cruciferous vegetables, all types of berries, onions, garlic, green tea, and ginger[119]. Plant-based protein does not hyper-activate TOR, since plants do not contain as much of the amino acid leucine as dairy and meat products do[120].

As to red meats, here's the latest from the United Nations World Health Organization's IARC (International Agency for Research on Cancer) as of October 26, 2015. In the IARC's Press Release No. 240, they declared red meat *"probably carcinogenic to humans (Group 2A)"* and processed meat was classified as *"carcinogenic to humans (Group 1)"*[121].

IARC also stated that *"The experts concluded that each 50 gram portion of processed meat eaten daily increases the risk of colorectal cancer by 18%."* "Red meat refers to all types of mammalian muscle meat, such as

---

119 http://www.ncbi.nlm.nih.gov/pmc/articles/PMC3711071/   accessed 1-7-2016
120 http://nutritionfacts.org/2015/06/16/living-longer-by-reducing-leucine-intake/ accessed 1-7-2016
121 https://www.iarc.fr/en/media-centre/pr/2015/pdfs/pr240_E.pdf accessed 1-7-2016

beef, veal, pork, lamb, mutton, horse, and goat." "Examples of processed meat include hot dogs (frankfurters), ham, sausages, corned beef, and biltong or beef jerky as well as canned meat and meat-based preparations and sauces." However, in my opinion, the IARC apparently overlooked mentioning delicatessen and sandwich meats, which are processed meats.

In order to prevent cancer, I think one of the most reasonable approaches would be to eat a diet that would be similar to what one would eat to beat cancer—a diet rich in antioxidants. Some of the best dietary sources of antioxidants, along with vitamin C, are colorful fruits and vegetables, e.g., broccoli, Brussel sprouts, cabbage, cauliflower, kale, mustard greens, parsley, hot and sweet bell peppers, raspberries, Romaine lettuce, tomatoes, watercress, and watermelon. I like to think of it as "eating a rainbow of color."

One of the most important and effective dietary regimens for any cancer patient is green tea. Green tea contains EGCG[122] (epigallocatechin-3-gallate) that has been shown to destroy cancer cells. According to the 2015 study, EGCG disrupts cancer cells mitochondria – the power house of all cells – by causing mitochondrial damage and the inability for cancer cells to function. Furthermore, that study also confirmed that EGCG did not damage normal healthy cells.

Vitamin C plays such an important role in beating cancer that recently it finally has been recognized as an effective treatment for cancer patients to be given intravenously[123]-[124]. There's a 2015 published paper "Metabolomic alterations in human cancer cells by vitamin C-induced oxidative stress" confirming *"that vitamin C inhibited energy metabolism through NAD* [Nicotinamide adenine dinucleotide, a co-enzyme in living cells] *depletion,*

---

122 http://www.ncbi.nlm.nih.gov/pubmed/25329972 accessed 3-7-20
123 http://www.ncbi.nlm.nih.gov/pubmed/26350063 accessed 2-20-16
124 http://www.ncbi.nlm.nih.gov/pmc/articles/PMC1405876/ accessed 2-20-16

thereby inducing cancer cell death."[125-126] Holistic medical doctors have been treating and managing cancer with mega dose vitamin C IVs for years!

Probably the best information regarding diet for beating cancer is found in the 23 chapters of Part II in my 2012 book *A Cancer Answer, Holistic BREAST Cancer Management, A Guide to Effective & Non-Toxic Treatments*, which is available on Amazon.com. It's the protocol I designed and used.

Cancer, unfortunately, is systemic and any type of cancer ought to respond to the diet in *A Cancer Answer*. Many women have used it with the same positive results, even to the amazement of their oncologists.

Skin cancer, once surgically removed, ought to be treated with a life-long cancer-prevention diet in order to preclude more skin cancers down the line.

Resources

Cancer Step Outside the Box
Author: Ty Bollinger
Publisher: Infinity 510 Partners / www.CancerTruth.net available on Amazon.com
ISBN 0-9788065-0-6

Recaging the Beast, The Disease Behind Disease: The Yeast-Fungal Connection
Author: Jane Remington
Publisher: Aerie LLC available on Amazon.com
ISBN 978-1-479-31847-6

---

[125] http://www.ncbi.nlm.nih.gov/pubmed/26350063 accessed 3-7-16
[126] http://www.ncbi.nlm.nih.gov/pmc/articles/PMC1405876/ accessed 3-7-16

HPV Vaccine Reactions: What can someone expect from diet and nutrition?

Ever since the HPV (human papillomavirus) vaccine came on the market in 2006—Gardasil®, the first to get FDA approval and licensure in the USA—thousands of young girls and women have experienced horrendous adverse side effects; some even fatal! Boys, starting around 9 years of age, take the HPV vaccines and they, too, have had adverse reactions.

SaneVax[127] is a consumer-health-oriented, international vaccine safety advocacy group whose mission is *"to promote only Safe, Affordable, Necessary & Effective vaccines and vaccination practices through education and information."* They believe in science-based medicine. Their primary goal is to provide the information necessary for healthcare consumers to make informed decisions regarding their health and wellbeing.

SaneVax also provides referrals to helpful resources for those unfortunate enough to have experienced vaccine-related injuries. Their website provides updates from the U.S. CDC/FDA VAERS reports for adverse reactions reported, including deaths, filed as official

---

127 http://sanevax.org/media-about/who/ accessed 12-21-15

reports with VAERS (Vaccine Adverse Event Reporting System). For those vaccinees, who have experienced adverse events and don't know that you and/or your physician should report them, there's an online reporting system you can use at https://vaers.hhs.gov/esub/index.

The last reporting numbers from VAERS listed by SaneVax, when I was writing this book, were taken from the VAERS March 2016 information, which stated 43,318 HPV vaccine adverse events, including 255 deaths. However, there were numerous other classifications like "Emergency Room 13,158" plus others, which I encourage you to read at the SaneVax website for the latest up-to-date CDC reporting numbers.

I bring up this topic of adverse reactions to the HPV vaccines, in particular, because vaccines per se are notoriously unsafe and not tested for their abilities to cause cancer, interfere with one's fertility, or cause birth defects in a growing fetus of a pregnant mother. Furthermore and globally, scores of young women have had their lives changed dramatically and negatively *forever* after receiving the HPV vaccines (Gardasil®, Cervarix®, and Gardasil 9®). However, there is a theory that there may be some relief available from the effects of histamine levels and releases in the body by restricting certain foods.

Cynthia A Janak, who researched the effects of histamine reactions[128] in girls reporting adverse events to the HPV vaccine, feels that since L-Histidine, which is a unique ingredient to the Gardasil® vaccines[129], just may precipitate an IgE release from it, thereby causing adverse reactions from excess histamine that, in turn, causes excess

---

128 http://healthimpactnews.com/2015/vaccine-mechanism-of-harm-exposed-in-gardasil/ accessed 12-21-15

129 http://www.fda.gov/downloads/BiologicsBloodVaccines/Vaccines/ApprovedProducts/UCM111263.pdf, pg. 12 accessed 12-21-15

inflammation in the body. Can there be histamine intolerance, which causes adverse reactions, in some people who receive vaccines? Very possibly!

Following her theory, Janak offers that foods containing histamine may exacerbate HPV-vaccine-injured-vaccinees' numerous recurring reactions. Janak suggests that HPV-damaged-vaccinees ought to structure their diets to avoid such foods as much as possible. With that in mind, I list Janak's suggestions[130] for a histamine-free diet.

One caveat Janak doesn't list regarding food, but I feel indispensable to regaining health, is absolutely no genetically-modified 'phoods' should be eaten and to maintain an organically-grown diet, since many crops can be sprayed pre-harvest with dangerous glyphosate[131].

Low histamine level foods:

- Fresh meat (cooled, frozen, or fresh)
- Freshly caught fish
- Chicken (skinned and fresh)
- Egg yolk
- Fresh fruits – with the exception of strawberries, most fresh fruits are considered to have a low histamine level (also see histamine liberators below)
- Fresh vegetables – with the exception of tomatoes
- Grains – rice noodles, yeast free rye bread, rice crisp bread, oats, puffed rice crackers, millet flour, pasta (spelt and corn based)
- Fresh pasteurized milk and milk products
- Milk substitutes – coconut milk, rice milk

---

130 Permission granted
131 http://www.ncbi.nlm.nih.gov/pubmed/15862083 accessed 2-18-16

- Cream cheese, butter (without the histamine generating rancidity)
- Most cooking oils – check suitability before use
- Most leafy herbs – check suitability before use
- Most non-citric fruit juices
- Herbal teas – with the exception of those listed below

High Level Histamine Foods:

Alcohol
Pickled or canned foods, e.g., sauerkrauts
Matured cheeses
Smoked meats, e.g., salami, ham, sausages
Shellfish
Beans and pulses, e.g., chickpeas, soy beans, peanuts
Nuts: walnuts, cashew nuts
Chocolates and other cocoa based products
Most citric fruits
Wheat based products
Vinegar
Ready meals
Salty snacks, sweets with preservatives and artificial colorings

Histamine Liberators:

Most citric fruits – kiwi, lemon, lime, pineapple, plums
Cocoa and chocolate
Nuts
Papaya
Beans and pulses
Tomatoes

Wheat germ
Additives: benzoate, sulphites, [nitrates], nitrites, glutamate [MSG], food dyes [colors]
Egg white only when in its raw state

Here's a more detailed listing of histamine foods[132] to avoid if you feel you may be or are histamine intolerant, a health condition most physicians still aren't very familiar with treating.

Fermented dairy products such as aged cheese, yogurt, and quark
Fermented or pickled vegetables
Tinned/canned, cured, and processed meats
Fermented soya products including miso, tempeh, and soy sauce
Green tea, matcha tea, coffee, cocoa, chocolate
All legumes (includes peanuts), and tree nuts (regular nuts)
Citrus fruits, raspberries, strawberries, bananas, pineapple, grapes, pears, and fruit juice
Avocado, eggplant, spinach, olives, tomato and tomato products (ketchup, tomato juice)
Vinegar, bouillon, and broth
Any alcohol
Junk foods or drinks that contain artificial colors or flavors

Personally, I think Janak's suggestions about foods' ability to affect histidine reactions probably should be taken seriously for their capability to exacerbate acute or chronic HPV vaccines adverse reactions. I further think, and suggest, histamine food interactions probably should be considered by anyone on the Autism Spectrum Disorder (ASD) and persons experiencing adverse reactions to any vaccines or vaccinations, no matter how long the endurance, e.g., several years or recent.

---

132 http://www.dietvsdisease.org/histamine-intolerance/ accessed 3-10-16

Additionally, as with all human exposures, allergic reactions can occur to histamines in food. About one percent of the population experiences adverse reactions to histamine in food, a problem which is overlooked but easy to diagnose[133] and treat. Histamine intolerance affects the integrity of the immune system.

---

133 http://theceliacmd.com/2014/03/histamine-intolerance-causing-symptoms/ accessed 3-10-16

Enzymes, Powerful 'Sparkplugs' in Food

What does a sparkplug do in the engine of your car? According to *Wikipedia*, a sparkplug *"is a device for delivering electric current from an ignition system to the combustion chamber of a spark-ignition engine to ignite the compressed fuel/air mixture by an electric spark, while containing combustion pressure within the engine."* In other words, delivering the power the engine needs!

Now, let's transfer that explanation, using the analogy format, to raw food enzymes. Enzymes are various proteins that act as catalysts for special biochemical actions within body chemistry, which I like to say are like "keys" that open doors to allow foods' life force nutrients into cells to do their work. That's why there's the popular raw food diet, which, unfortunately, some folks can't tolerate for numerous reasons.

My thinking on raw food diets is that they are paramount in fighting and beating cancer! Dr Max Gerson, MD, proved that time and again. Eating to beat cancer means eating as much as 75 to 80 percent of your diet as raw, organically-grown foods—no animal products at all! Many holistic cancer protocols include numerous enzyme supplements too.

However, there's the macrobiotic approach to cancer, which for many years was a totally cooked diet that really worked!

Personally, as a cancer survivor and retired *natural* nutritionist, who dealt with thousands of clients, I can attest to the fact that when clients changed their diets from the modern western junk food diets to a plant-based diet, everyone got well—some even went off disability and back to work!

As an aside, my stint with breast cancer can be attributed not to a nondiscretionary diet, which has been clean and plant-based since the 1970s, but from being exposed to formaldehyde in the 1970s; a neighbor who for 13 years sprayed Roundup® almost weekly in the garden just over the fence from ours; and some unscrupulous individuals cooking what officials thought may have been "meth" and venting fumes somewhere in the neighborhood. But, I'm still here and cancer free—thank God! You may be interested in the book I wrote *A Cancer Answer, Holistic BREAST Cancer Management* while working my all holistic protocol to deal with breast cancer. The book is available on Amazon.com.

Air, water, and food are the major resources upon which the human body runs. A body can die without any or all of those three depending upon varying circumstances. There's no getting away from it: we must feed our bodies the way Nature intended or else we will become dis-eased.

Nevertheless, if you prepare your foods using low heat and organically-grown produce that is still crunchy or *a la dente*, as the recipes in this book advise, you can maintain most, if not all, of the food values and enzymes, which are keys to rebuilding health and maintaining it. However, some foods like cabbage family vegetables and spinach actually need to be heated for better bioavailability—mushrooms too.

It's important to have a diet rich in magnesium, which most berries provide generously, because the mineral magnesium is involved in over 300 enzyme reactions! Our bodies manufacture enzymes; we can get enzymes from supplements; but, the best source of enzymes is raw, organically-grown food.

If you experience any of the following symptoms, you probably need more enzymes (water and fiber) in your diet:

- Acid reflux or heartburn
- Bloating and/or abdominal distension at times, especially a few hours after eating a meal
- Burping or belching
- Constipation
- Flatulence—passing gas; farting

Dr Tim O'Shea, DC, feels enzymes are the key to longevity. One of his comments fits in with the above:

"The pain is commonly described as a burning. The chronic situation that ensues typically involves the gut mucosa, from the esophagus all the way on down. Chronic inflammation, coupled with digestive enzyme depletion – all this brings on pain."

The foods that are known specifically for their enzymes are:

Papaya contains the proteolytic enzyme papain. Papaya makes a wonderful snack or breakfast fruit all by itself with fresh lime juice sprinkled all over.

Pineapple contains cysteine proteinase for digesting proteins. Bromelain in pineapple is an effective anti-inflammatory enzyme!

Bee pollen contains a 'laundry list' of enzymes: amylase, catalase, cozymase, cytochrome, dehydrogenase, diaphorase, diastase, pectase, and phosphatase.

Fermented vegetables include Kimchee, sauerkraut and fermented: cabbage, carrots, cucumbers, eggplant, onions, and squash.

Other foods with high enzyme content include: avocado, buttermilk, coconut water, grapes, raw pure local honey, kefir (a fermented dairy milk-like drink), kiwi, mango, melons, and wheat grass juice.

However, all raw foods contain enzymes; they come "built in" for helping the body to digest food.

To give you an idea of how raw food enzymes work, let's consider making a jelled dessert like Jell-O™ adding pineapple to lime Jell-O™. The package directions will tell you to use drained canned pineapple, not fresh! Why? The enzymes! Raw pineapple enzymes will not allow the Jell-O™ to set and jell; they will keep it liquid. However, canned pineapple is high heat treated in canning and destroys those raw enzymes and will not interfere with the jelling of animal byproducts from which gelatin is made. Gelatin is a dehydrated protein byproduct made by boiling animal skins, tendons, ligaments, and/or bones with water, packaged with proprietary ingredients and sold as a dessert. Remember, pineapple contains cysteine proteinase for digesting proteins. See how enzymes work?

One easy way to make certain you get plenty of fresh food enzymes in your daily diet is to incorporate sprouts[134] and microgreens like watercress. Alfalfa, arugula, broccoli, buckwheat, clover, fenugreek, mung beans, radish, sunflower, or any mixture of sprouts, can be added as gar-

---

134   http://www.superfoods-for-superhealth.com/super-sprouts.html   accessed 1-31-16

nishes to entrées, soups and stews, open face sandwiches, and definitely include sprouts on top of leafy green salads.

Another excellent source of fresh plant-based enzymes is wheat grass juice, plus all freshly-pressed fruit and vegetable juices. One caution, though, that I would like to share. I suggest keeping fruit and their juices to themselves and not combine them with vegetables, grains, or animal products if you eat meat, dairy, cheese, and eggs. Fruit enzymes pass through the digestive tract very quickly and don't allow enough time in the stomach for proteins, starches, and sugars in more complex foods eaten with fruit to be mixed with gastric juices in the stomach before passing into the small intestines where digestive problems can occur along with what's called "leaky gut," which exacerbates all types of digestive and chronic disease issues. It's called "proper food combinations[135]," which can be rather difficult to accept and to follow when one eats a standard American diet. Eat fruit 30 minutes before other food, except nuts, or 2 hours after eating carbs, fats, and proteins for proper food combining.

However, I'm convinced about many aspects of food combining since I found it to be the only thing to work with clients who had difficult digestive problems. Once they were fed up with being sick and changed to proper food combinations, they improved almost immediately and said they would stick with it forever. Nothing works like first-hand experience, I guess. I share that because today's nutrition information considers proper food combining to be "quackery." However, when it works, who's to condemn it then?

Not to stray too far off topic, I'd like to point out that our pets, dogs in particular, are coming down with arthritis, cancers, and other chronic diseases[136] which, I offer, are due in part to the diet we feed them, es-

---

[135] http://www.acidalkalinediet.net/correct-food-combining-principles.php accessed 1-31-16
[136] http://www.embracepetinsurance.com/coverage/chronic-conditions accessed 1-31-16

pecially dry dog chow! Veterinarians are offering similar health services as physicians provide for people with chronic diseases! Partially, it's the food, I contend. All pet foods contain GMOs, unless you purchase organically-produced dog[137] and cat[138] food, or make your own[139].

Another example of diet causing problems, I contend, is found in dairy cows who are fed GMO feed (alfalfa, corn, and soy) which, as ruminant animals, cows were intended by Nature to eat the grasses of the fields and prairies, not be prisoned in barns and fed GMOs at food troughs, plus being injected with genetically engineered growth hormones (rBST and rBGH) to produce more milk. As a result, cows can end up with mastitis of the udder and have to be given antibiotics to clear up the infection, in addition to the other pharmaceutical drugs put into factory-farmed animal feed.

Cows and all ruminant animals are supposed to be grass-fed and browsers—out in the open fields—not trying to digest corn and soy bean starches which, I think, makes cows produce more burping, cow farts, and methane [140].

Not only do we get enzymes in our food, but our body manufactures them too: the salivary glands, stomach, pancreas, liver, and small intestine. That's why it's so extremely important to chew foods very well—at least 20 times in order to insalivate it—before swallowing.

Did you know that 90 percent of digestion and absorption takes place in the small intestines? If you experience discomfort in the center of your abdomen in the area around your belly button, that

---

137   http://www.organic-pet-digest.com/10-best-dog-food-options.html accessed 2-17-16
138   http://www.onlynaturalpet.com/search/cats/food/organic-foods?click=55&gclid=CIPQ5sDL_8oC FYcYHwodTjcCng accessed 2-17-16
139   http://www.moneycrashers.com/homemade-dog-food-treat-recipes/ accessed 2-17-16
140   http://scienceline.ucsb.edu/getkey.php?key=2569 accessed 1-31-16

could be an indication that you are having digestive problems in the small intestine.

If you experience a lot of burping and flatulence, what does that have to say about your digestive processes?

The Incredible, Edible B-complex Vitamins: The nutritional enzyme system enablers for cell metabolism

All nutrients are important in human physiology, but the B-complex vitamins have a very special place in this *natural* nutritionist's heart and consciousness. Why? Because they are needed by all body systems but, unfortunately, are grossly lacking in today's modern food culture due to processed foods and our penchant for fast and junk foods, plus the lack of a diversified plant-based diet.

B-complex vitamins are "water soluble," extremely fragile, and can be destroyed by milling grains, food processing techniques, evaporation, soaking, cooking, oxidation—even microwave cooking can destroy B-12. B-complex vitamins are easily excreted from the body, too. Furthermore, since they function as coenzymes to help the body extract and retain energy from foods, it's paramount to optimum health that they be present in our foods and diet on a continual and daily basis.

Here are food sources of B vitamins:

Thiamine B1: Black beans, barley, broccoli, dried peas, green peas, lentils, lima beans, navy beans, oats, pinto beans, sunflower seeds

Riboflavin B2: Almonds, asparagus, beet greens, Cremini mushrooms, cherries, collard greens, soy beans, spinach, turnip greens

Niacin B3: Avocado, brown rice, fresh green peas, Portobello mushrooms, sunflower seeds

Pantothenic Acid B5: Avocado, mushrooms: brown, Chanterelle, Oyster, Portobello, Shiitake, white, sunflower seeds, sweet potatoes

Pyridoxine B6: Pearl barley, broccoli, Brussel sprouts, brown rice, carrots, cauliflower, corn, Great Northern beans, kidney beans, lentils, lima beans, peas, potato, soybeans, spinach, sunflower seeds, tomatoes

Biotin B7: Almonds, avocado, banana, broccoli, brown rice, cabbage, cauliflower, green peas, lentils, oats, pecans, peanuts, raspberries, soybeans, split peas, spinach, strawberries, walnuts

Folate B9: Asparagus, banana, pearled barley, beets, broccoli, Brussel sprouts, cabbage, carrots, cauliflower, chick peas, cowpeas, grapefruit, green beans, kale, lima beans, orange, peas, pinto beans, potato, Romaine lettuce, soybeans, spinach, tomato

Cobalamin B12: Animal meats and foods, soy tempeh, fortified soy products, nutrition supplements, and vitamin-mineral pills

As vitamin B-complex "insurance," daily I take a natural B-complex vitamin capsule made from *organically-grown foods sources*—not synthetics—once in the morning and again after dinner.

However, I also eat a diet rich in vitamin B-complex foods. Do you?

The Energy Vitamins Everyone Overlooks

One of the most shameful nutritional adverse side effects of processed foods, in my opinion as a *natural* nutritionist, is the fact that many, if not all fast food menus and munchies we love to gnash on, are highly deficient in B-complex vitamins—what are called the "energy" vitamins. So, what are the B-complex vitamins, and why are they critically important to human health and wellbeing?

First of all, the B's are water soluble—as opposed to fat soluble, which means they are "self-regulating," don't store in the body, and pass through the body via urination if and when we get too many of any one of them at any time. The other "twist" about the B vitamins is that humans must take the entire B-complex in supplementation form (capsule or powder) in order to get a *pharmacological-like effect* of any one specific B vitamin like B-6 or B-12 to nutritionally impact nerve pain/damage or anemia.

The B-complex roster, which most researchers consider as the complex, includes: thiamine (vitamin B1), riboflavin (vitamin B2), niacin (vitamin B3), choline (vitamin B4), pantothenic acid (vitamin B5), pyridoxine (vitamin B6), biotin (vitamin B7), inositol (vitamin B8), folic acid (vitamin B9) and PABA [Para-aminobenzoic acid] (vitamin B10), and the cobalamins (vitamin B12). However, there are a few other B vitamins that are not promoted, but still appear in the scientific literature and are used by some practitioners, which I list below.

Just to impress the importance of the various B-complex vitamins and how they work with body chemistry, here is an abbreviated summary of what specific B vitamins provide and do with biochemistry, besides helping all enzyme systems to work efficiently:

B-1	Carbohydrate metabolism, nervous system function, appetite control
B-2	Energy metabolism, metabolism of carbohydrates, fats, and proteins
B-3	Needed for almost all the body's metabolic processes, metabolism of carbohydrates, fats, and proteins
B-4	*aka* Choline: Metabolism of fats and cholesterol; formation of DNA and RNA; muscle, nerve and memory function; needed for manganese metabolism; and is a B-complex co-factor
B-5	Energy metabolism; hormone formation; metabolism of energy from fats and carbs
B-6	Acts as a co-enzyme involved with metabolism; it's needed to process the minerals magnesium, manganese and zinc; and to process many essential fatty acids (EFAs) and many of the amino acids
B-7	*aka* Biotin: Actually can be manufactured by a *healthy* gut/microbiome/intestinal tract; necessary for carbohydrate, fat, and protein metabolism
B-8	Gene expression; breakdown of fats; insulin signal transduction; cell membrane maintenance
B-9	Necessary for the formation of blood and antibodies; needed for cell division and the metabolism of sugars and amino acids

B-10	PABA: an effective sun screen; co-factor of the B-complex; needed in the formation of folic acid
B-11	Pteryl-hepta-glutamic acid, a form of folic acid needed by humans
B-12	Production of red blood cells; fat and protein metabolism; create and maintain cell membranes
B-16	Dimethylglycine is synthesized in the human body from choline (B-4)
B-17	Nitrilosides / Amygdalin / Laetrile: Controversial vitamin obtained from plant source seeds used in the holistic treatment and management of cancer

One Internet online seller of B-complex vitamins[141] provides a handy, dandy list of which ones in the B-complex vitamins can be used for certain health conditions and the reasoning behind the recommendations. Please know, and be assured, that I have no affiliation of any type with *eVitamins*, I'm just passing along information for whatever it may be worth, as with all the information I share.

However, and here's my caveat, many B-complex vitamin supplements are synthetically manufactured and are not as bioavailable as they could or should be, especially if someone has either digestive or intestinal health problems. That's where the flora, or microbiome of the gut, is so extremely important in regaining—and the maintenance of—health and wellbeing, especially the quantitative and qualitative status of B-complex vitamins within your body. To understand more, please refer to the *What Goes In Must Come Out: A necessary discussion about poop* to appreciate more fully the importance of gut health, including the role B-complex vitamins play in microbiome population and production, human health, and maintaining the body's defense system

---

141 http://www.evitamins.com/encyclopedia/assets/nutritional-supplement/vitamin-b-complex/~default accessed 2-15-16

against diseases—the immune system, which "resides" within the intestinal tract.

What happens to those precious B-complex vitamins during food processing?

Quite frankly, many if not most, can be destroyed by any or all of the following:

1. Transportation: Food that has to travel far and long can experience evaporation of water soluble B-complex vitamins, especially leafy greens.
2. Food stored in hot warehouses and hot cars, which also can turn fats in food rancid!
3. Paring, peeling, or winnowing of outer fiber coatings of grains (rice, wheat), fruits, and vegetables.
4. High-heat processing for canned foods, which can destroy B vitamins due to their being heat-labile. As an example, "heat labile protein" is protein that changed or was nutritionally damaged by high heat temperatures during cooking or processing.
5. Very little *real food ingredients* are in processed snack and junk foods. Read ingredient labels to realize all the chemicals that are added at low manufacturing costs to make a market-profitable "edible." Without real food, there's very little likelihood of real nutrients in it! That's why many synthetic vitamins have to be added to some "raw products" like wheat flour. That flour by law has to be "enriched" with four synthetic vitamins and one mineral, because during the processing of wheat kernels, eleven vitamins and one mineral are removed, therefore most wheat flours are nutritionally deficient. Similar processing happens with rice, which then has to be enriched or "fortified." During processing, rice loses the mineral iron, and these B vitamins:

Thiamine (B1), Niacin (B3) and Folic acid (B9), which are added back by chemical synthetics.
6. However, during the winnowing of grains, the nutritionally valuable outer coating, where the B vitamins reside, is stripped away leaving starchy flours that do not have all the components Nature supplied for grains to be digested and metabolically processed properly in the human gut, thereby making starchy carbs turn into a fat-producing-sugars in the body. Now, can you understand why junk food makes people fat?

It is my opinion that the most bioavailable way to ingest and biochemically process B-complex vitamins is by eating a whole foods, plant-based, organically- and sustainably-grown diet. That, for some individuals, may not be as easy as it sounds—and because of various reasons—the least of which is changing from the SAD—standard American diet—to a NEW—nutritionally energized wholefoods—food shopping, preparing, cooking, and eating lifestyle.

Even though I profess and practice as close to a one-hundred-percent plant-based food plan, I understand that others still will want to eat *nutritious, humanely-grown, grass-fed* animal products. If that be the case, I would encourage that animal-based food be 20 percent, or less, of your diet. Organically-grown, non-GMO whole grains, beans, legumes, nuts, fresh fruit, and vegetables should make up the balance—80 percent.

So, what are the foods that supply substantial amounts of the B-complex vitamins?

B-1 Thiamine
Animal sources: ham, pork, salmon
Plant food sources: almonds, beans, berries, dark leafy green vegetables, flax seeds, green peas, lentils, wheat germ, whole grain

cereals and baked goods, pecans, soy foods—tofu, sunflower seeds

B-2 Riboflavin
Animal sources: dairy products like cheese, milk and yogurt, chicken, eggs, fish, turkey
Plant food sources: asparagus, broccoli, leafy greens, mushrooms, nuts, spinach, whole grains

B-3 Niacin
Animal sources: chicken, eggs, salmon, tuna, turkey
Plant food sources: legumes, peanuts, nutritional yeast, whole wheat

B-5 Pantothenic acid
Animal sources: organ meats, salmon, yogurt
Plant food sources: avocados, broccoli, legumes, lentils, mushrooms, split peas, sweet potatoes

B-6 Pyridoxine
Animal sources: eggs, poultry, red meat, salmon, seafood
Plant food sources: avocado, bananas, beans, green beans, leafy greens, e.g., spinach, lentils, potatoes, sunflower seeds, sweet potatoes, walnuts

B-7 Biotin
Animal sources: cheese, egg yolk, liver, pork, organ meats, salmon
Plant food sources: avocado, most fruits and vegetables, whole grains

B-9 Folate / Folic acid
Animal sources: pork, poultry

Plant food sources: asparagus, beans, Brussel sprouts, citrus fruits, leafy greens, lentils, parsnips, red beets, spinach, tomato juice, turnip greens, whole grains

B-12 Cobalamins
Animal sources: beef, eggs, fin fish, milk and dairy products, salmon, shell fish
Plant food sources: yeast extract; *possibly in certain algae*, e.g., [*Porphyra yezoensis* (Nori)], [*Palmaria palmate* (Dulse)], Kelp, Kombu, and Wakame; *very little in some mushrooms*: Black Trumpet, Golden chanterelle, Porcini, Oyster, Black Morels

Please Note: For those who maintain a vegan diet, or a diet that has very little animal foods, a B-12 vitamin supplement should be taken to prevent vitamin B-12 deficiency diseases. However, a healthy gut microbiome can produce some vitamins, e.g., B-12, thiamine, riboflavin, and vitamin K. Vitamin B-12 deficiency can lead to anemia, nerve and brain damage, and pernicious anemia. Tiredness and heart palpitations can be a sign of a vitamin B-12 deficiency, especially anemia. In elderly folks, there's the risk of brain shrinkage due to lack of B-12.

The B-complex vitamins are more important than you probably realized. They, unfortunately, are the nutrients most easily damaged or depleted by modern food processing techniques, fast food menus, high-heat food preparation, plus eating a diet based in starchy carbohydrates, munchies, and snacks out of packages or boxes.

Hopefully, my thumbnail explanation about the nutritional importance of the B-complex vitamins will turn you on to eating whole plant-based foods, and turn you off from eating junk foods and snacks.

An exceptional plant food vitamin B-packed snack, in my opinion, is an organically grown ripe banana with a handful or two of raw pecans, walnuts, or sunflower seeds. Some organic Trail Mixes contain a respectable assortment of dried fruits and raw nuts that provide a nice complement of B vitamins, provided some of the ingredients aren't sweetened with sugars or coated with rancid oils.

B-complex Vitamins in
Foods That Are Enablers for Cell Metabolism

B1 Thiamine
Black beans, barley, dried peas, green peas, lentils, lima beans, Navy beans, oats, Pinto beans, sunflower seeds

B2 Riboflavin
Almonds, asparagus, beet greens, Cremini mushrooms, broccoli, cherries, collard greens, soy beans, spinach, turnip greens

B3 Niacin
Avocado, brown rice, fresh green peas, Portobello mushrooms, sunflower seeds

B5 Pantothenic Acid
Avocado, mushrooms: Brown, Chanterelle, Oyster, Portobello, Shiitake, White, sunflower seeds, sweet potatoes

B6 Pyridoxine
Pearl barley, broccoli, Brussel sprouts, brown rice, carrots, cauliflower, corn, Great Northern beans, kidney beans, lentils, lima beans, peas, potato, soybeans, spinach, sunflower seeds, tomatoes

B7 Biotin
Almonds, avocado, banana, broccoli, brown rice, cabbage, cauliflower, oats, peanuts, green peas, split peas, pecans, raspberries, soybeans, spinach, strawberries, walnuts

B9 Folate (Folic Acid)
Asparagus, banana, pearled barley, beets, broccoli, Brussel sprouts, cabbage, carrots, cauliflower, chick peas, cowpeas, grapefruit, green beans, kale, lima beans, orange, peas, pinto beans, potato, Romaine lettuce, soybeans, spinach, tomato

B12 Cobalamin
Soy tempeh, fortified soy products, nutritional supplements

Fermented Foods: What do they have to do with maintaining good health?

If you like sauerkraut, you are familiar with the concept of fermented foods. However, most commercially-produced sauerkrauts leave much to be desired, in my humble opinion. Why? Well, the ingredients, for one thing, and the method of fermentation for another.

Fermented foods are all about providing living organisms that feed and enhance our gut, or the microbiome, flora. Those organisms aid in digestion and assimilation thereby providing maximum nutrition from food to support our immune system due to the lactic acid they produce. Plus, they taste wonderful, too!

So, what kind of fermented foods are there? There's a wide variety from plant-based foods:

Fermented tofu
Kimchi (a Korean condiment made with cabbage and spices)
Kombucha (a form of fermented tea)
Miso (a Japanese style paste-like culinary ingredient)

Natto (a traditional Japanese soy recipe prized for its enzyme, Nattokinase)
Onions
Pickled beets (my all-time favorite)
Pickled cabbage
Pickled carrots
Pickled corn and corn relish
Pickled cucumbers
Pickled garlic
Pickled radish
Sauerkraut
Sour pickles
Soy sauce
Tempeh (fermented soy)
Turnips

Then, there are animal-source fermented foods such as yogurt, buttermilk, kefir (a milk-based fermented beverage), Lassi (a delicious Indian cuisine yogurt beverage), and some fermented cottage cheese.

Learning how to make your own fermented foods is very easy. There are many online resources to guide you in preparing these no-cook, fermented foods[142].

People have been making fermented foods for ages. Even in Roman times they had sauerkraut! The key ingredient in making fermented foods is salt, which precipitates a naturally-occurring breakdown of the raw food that invites ambient airborne microbes (bacteria) to join in the action. During the breakdown, healthful lactic acid and enzymes are produced, which give fermented foods their deliciously unique tastes, textures, and healthful immune system enhancing nutrients.

---
142 http://articles.mercola.com/sites/articles/archive/2012/12/15/caroline-barringer-interview.aspx accessed 3-5-16

Miso is a fermented bean or grain seasoning that is added mainly to soups, but can be added to sauces and other dishes too. It can be made from grain (barley, millet, rice) or beans (chick peas, yellow and black soy beans). I prefer garbanzo bean miso since, basically, it's neutral for everyone (gluten-free), plus it's exceptionally tasty too.

Miso's health properties include that it can protect against harmful radiation; boosts the immune system; guards against intestinal diseases, including cancer; and soy isoflavones in miso made from soybeans, according to the Japan Public Health Center-Based Prospective Study on Cancer and Cardiovascular Diseases[143], are effective in preventing breast cancer.

However, there is a caveat about fermented foods for certain people. If you are histamine intolerant, then histamine foods like miso and fermented foods listed above should be eliminated from your diet. There is a blood test to determine if you are histamine intolerant. It's called the Histamine Intolerance Test, and it may be an answer to prayer if you've been having gastrointestinal health problems that can't seem to be resolved. More information about that test can be found at this website[144] http://www.lsialab.com/gb/histamine_intolerance_test.

Resources
How to Easily and Inexpensively Ferment Your Own Vegetables
http://articles.mercola.com/sites/articles/archive/2012/12/15/caroline-barringer-interview.aspx

Immunitrition Cultured Vegetables Online Store
http://www.culturedvegetables.net/Cultured-Vegetables_c3.htm

---

143 http://epi.ncc.go.jp/en/jphc/248/87.html accessed 3-10-16
144 http://www.lsialab.com/gb/histamine_intolerance_test accessed 3-10-15

About Miso, including how to cook with miso
http://www.southrivermiso.com/store/pg/63-About-Miso-Links/Resources.html

A Guide to Different Kinds of Miso and How to Use Them
http://www.huffingtonpost.com/2015/04/03/different-kinds-of-miso_n_6993590.html

Protein, the Building Blocks of Life

Every cell in our bodies contains and needs protein[145]. However, what you may not know is that there are about ten thousand different proteins, according to the Harvard School of Public Health, which help the human body to function. Furthermore, I contend, the type of protein (animal or plant), its source (organically or conventionally grown/produced), quantity (too much animal protein may be harmful, depending upon individual biochemistry), and *quality* (nutritional content and food preparation) probably are the most important factors in restoring and/or maintaining vibrant health.

Literally, we are what we eat!

Another apparently unknown factoid is almost all whole-raw foods humans eat contain some protein content, even vegetables! Generally speaking, there are approximately 2 to 3 grams of protein in every 100 grams of veggies eaten, including foods like white mushrooms and spinach. Beans and legumes, on the other hand, contain higher amounts—over 5 grams of vegetable protein per 100 grams eaten. However, *sprouted* beans, peas, and lentils contain as high as 13 grams of protein per 100 grams eaten.

---

145 http://myhome.sunyocc.edu/~weiskirl/amino_acids_proteins.htm accessed 12-15-15

But there's a *technicality* about protein! Even though there are 20 different amino acids, there are two basic classifications of protein: *complete,* which contains all 9 essential amino acids[146], and *incomplete,* which lack the full chain of essential amino acids and must be combined correctly to make a complete amino acid chain of protein.

Before we get too involved with protein, here are those 20 amino acids:

Alanine Arginine Asparagine Aspartic Acid Cysteine Glutamine Glutamic Acid Glycine Histidine Isoleucine Leucine Lysine Methionine Phenylalanine Proline Serine Threonine Tryptophan Tyrosine Valine

The 9 *essential* amino acids are:

Histidine Isoleucine Leucine Lysine Methionine
Phenylalanine Threonine Tryptophan Valine

Regarding the other 11 amino acids, the trick to making a complete amino acid chain is found in the combinations of foods:

Beans and legumes (lentils, peanuts) combined with grains, i.e., rice, wheat, barley, etc. or dairy products
Grains with dairy products
Seeds (Sesame, sunflower, pumpkin) with beans and legumes

By the way, speaking of amino acids, there are two organic, gluten-free, non-GMO, and dairy-free liquid cooking seasonings that contain amino acids, which add more nutrition to recipes, while functioning in recipes similarly to soy sauce taste. One, which is soy based, is *Braggs Liquid Aminos All Purpose Seasoning from Soy Protein,* and the other, which is

---

146   https://en.wikipedia.org/wiki/Complete_protein accessed 12-15-15

coconut based, is *Coconut Secret Raw Coconut Aminos Soy-free Seasoning Sauce*. Braggs has a more traditional soy sauce taste, while Coconut Secret has a sweeter flavor, in my opinion. The sodium contents differ, so check that out in the event you are concerned about sodium. According to the Daily Values listing for sodium, a 2,000 calorie diet should have less than 2,400 mg of sodium a day; while a 2,500 calorie diet ought to have the same, less than 2,400 mg of sodium per day.

One exception to the incomplete plant-protein rule is the ancient Inca grain, *Quinoa*, actually a seed, I contend. It contains all amino acids that make a complete protein. Even though Quinoa has all the amino acids, it does not have them in sufficient quantity that would make it equivalent to animal-source complete protein.

Legumes, however, have higher amounts of incomplete proteins too.

A popular seed with quality vegetable protein is *Chia*. In one ounce, or 28 grams of chia seeds, there are 4 grams of protein, compared with 5 grams of protein for the same amount of flax seeds and a whopping 9 grams of protein for the same amount of hemp seeds.

By contrast, sesame seeds—even though very tasty when toasted and sprinkled on veggies, steamed rice, or soup—don't contain very much plant protein. One tablespoon of sesame seeds contains only 6.9 grams of plant protein.

Ezekiel Bread (health food store item) contains 8 grams of complete complementary proteins in 2 slices of delicious *sprouted* grain, seed, and legume bread. That bread is more nutritious and highly digestible due to the grains, seeds, and legumes having been sprouted and then made into bread flour. However delicious it is, *it still contains gluten*.

The fusion-style of cooking and eating takes into consideration varied cuisines from around the globe that provide excellent complementary-protein recipes. Here are some example dishes:

Asian: brown rice and soybeans; tofu and sesame seeds

Asian Indian: dal (lentils/beans) soup or stew and rice with Indian Lassi (yogurt drink); chickpea curry with Basmati rice

Latin American/Mexican: rice and beans; corn tortillas and beans; bean and cheese enchiladas

Macrobiotic diet: originated with the Japanese plant-based diet centered around brown rice, soy products, fresh and fermented vegetables, and seaweeds

Middle Eastern: hummus (chickpeas and tahini—sesame seed butter); chickpea and Basmati rice salad; falafel sandwich (chickpea 'meatballs' inside whole wheat pita bread with salad greens and a spicy sauce)

Vegan diet: fruits, grains, nuts, seeds, vegetables

Protein intake recommendations vary between 0.4 and 0.8 grams of protein per kilogram of body weight. One kilogram equals approximately 2.2 pounds. A 125 pound person's daily protein intake should approximate 23 grams of protein calculated at 0.4, but 45 grams of protein calculated at 0.8 grams.

It's important to know that older persons, e.g., senior citizens, plus vegans, probably should increase their intake above the 0.4 grams per kilogram—something like 0.6 grams of protein per kilogram of body weight. That same 125-pound person, if a senior citizen or vegan, then should be ingesting 34 grams of protein per day.

Here's how to figure what your daily consumption of protein in grams ought to be:

Your weight in pounds _____ divided by 2.2 = _____
x 0.4 = _____ daily protein grams

According to the U.S. Food and Drug Administration's "Guidance for Industry: A Food Labeling Guide," the guideline for Daily Value (DV) for protein is set at 50 grams for adults and children over 4 years of age[147]. If those 50 grams of protein are from animal sources, I venture to say that diabetes, cardiovascular, kidney diseases, cancer, and gout probably will become future health concerns.

However, if you'd like to calculate what your Body Mass Index (BMI) presently is, plus the correct range for your age and height, you may be interested in an online Internet site "How much should I weigh for my height and age?" at this URL address http://40plusstyle.com/how-much-should-i-weigh-for-my-height-and-age/comment-page-1/.

For folks who eat animal protein, I think there is some information you ought to know and consider seriously regarding the impact of red meat, in particular, on health, which may prompt your eating style to become "flexitarian"—meaning eating less red meat, less often – i.e., only two servings per week, but not completely eliminating it from your diet, while also making certain you choose the most healthful and "clean" cuts of red meat. Reduce animal dairy product consumption to only three hormone-free servings per week. Any eggs should be from

---

[147] http://www.fda.gov/Food/GuidanceRegulation/GuidanceDocumentsRegulatoryInformation/LabelingNutrition/ucm064928.htm accessed 12-16-15

pasture- or organically-raised hens. Personally, I have a problem with the cholesterol 'myth' associated with eggs, since a healthy human liver naturally produces between 2,000 and 3,000 milligrams of cholesterol a day for bone, hormones, and all life processes. The brain is full of cholesterol and even manufacturers some! Did you know that 25 percent of all cholesterol in your body is in your brain[148]?

According to *Prevention* on line, here are some pretty sensible reasons to stop eating red meat:

1. *"Eating red meat hardens blood vessels.*
2. *Your vegetarian friends may outlive you.*
3. *You're eating pink slime, aka lean finely textured beef.*
4. *That expensive filet may be 'glued' together meat scraps.*
5. *Livestock production impacts the planet in huge way. [And negatively too!]*
6. *You can get sick from E.coli.*
7. *The animal cruelty factor is sickening.*
8. *Eating meat ups the risk of type 2 diabetes.*
9. *Meat puts your colon and brain at risk.*
10. *Meat is chockful of harmful hormones."*[149]

So, exactly what hormones are likely to be in meat? There's recombinant bovine growth hormone (rBGH) injected into cows to produce more milk, which may increase the production of another naturally-occurring hormone in the body, insulin-like growth factor (IGF) that is implicated in human cancer formations; sex hormones given to cattle, estrogen (estradiol in particular), via an ear implant that also can contain other hormones[150] e.g., pituitary hormones like somatotropins. Then

---

148 http://www.drperlmutter.com/brain-needs-cholesterol/ accessed 12-15-15
149 http://www.prevention.com/food/healthy-eating-tips/10-reasons-to-stop-eating-red-meat accessed 12-15-15
150 http://www.merckvetmanual.com/mvm/pharmacology/growth_promotants_and_production_enhancers/steroid_hormones.html accessed 12-15-15

there's "Zeranol®, a non-steroidal estrogen agonist" that can increase cancer proliferation in existing breast cancer[151]. In livestock fattening feed lots, cattle are given Diethylstilbestrol (DES). Is there any wonder why 160 countries say "NO" to USA-produced meats?

The answer is because ractopamine, a synthetic beta-agonist drug, is given to cattle and pigs in the days leading up to slaughter, and that veterinary drug is banned in other countries[152]. There can be residues of that drug left in butchered meat! Another weight-producing, pre-slaughter beta-agonist drug is Zilmax®, which can add as much as 30 pounds of lean meat per cow[153]. Can or does eating those synthetic weight-producing-hormones in cattle also add weight to humans?

Hopefully, everyone can understand the merits of reducing or eliminating altogether conventionally-grown CAFO (confined animal feeding operations) meats, and really appreciate the healthful qualities of sustainably-grown, grass-fed, non-GMO, organically-produced animal meats, dairy products, and eggs.

The last piece of information I'd like to discuss about protein is "Are you protein deficient" and how to determine that, especially if you are vegan or vegetarian and aren't getting enough complete and complementary proteins in your diet.

Here are a few signs that you may be protein deficient:

1. Hair falling out
2. If you get weak after exercise or physical activity
3. Are you tired when you should not be?
4. Do you get injured easily and can't seem to recover easily?

---

151   https://en.wikipedia.org/wiki/Zeranol accessed 12-15-15
152   http://articles.mercola.com/sites/articles/archive/2013/12/24/ractopamine-beta-agonist-drug.aspx accessed 12-15-15
153   Ibid.

5. Nails and skin are not healthy looking or flabby
6. Overweight: That may be an indication of a junk-food-rich diet rather than a properly balanced, healthful diet with complex carbohydrates and complementary proteins. Many vegetarians inadvertently live off of "health food store junk foods," in my opinion.

To rectify a protein deficiency, there are protein powders and mixes, which I caution about using since they may contain toxic heavy metals, especially arsenic from rice proteins used to make them. The Health Ranger, Mike Adams, has tested many vegetarian protein powders, since he operates the Natural News Forensic Food Labs (http://labs.naturalnews.com/), which assays food to determine if toxic heavy metals are in them. Arsenic has been found in rice[154]. The article "Vegan protein powders with low heavy metals: Health Ranger reveals the cleanest products tested so far" at http://www.naturalnews.com/045108_vegan_proteins_heavy_metals_laboratory_test_results.html, explains what NNFFL found, and which I heartily recommend anyone interested in protein powders ought to check out.

---

154 http://www.consumerreports.org/cro/magazine/2015/01/how-much-arsenic-is-in-your-rice/index.htm accessed 12-16-15

Resources

The Best Protein Choices and Worst for Your Health and the Environment
http://www.eatingwell.com/food_news_origins/green_sustainable/best_meat_worst_meat_the_best_protein_choices

Meatless Monday
http://www.meatlessmonday.com/about-us/why-meatless/

Rain Crow Ranch Monthly Buying Club
http://www.americangrassfedbeef.com/grass-fed-beef-roasts.asp
http://www.americangrassfedbeef.com/monthly-grass-fed-beef.asp

Eatwild's Directory of U.S., Canadian and International Farms and Ranches
http://www.eatwild.com/products/

Thrive Market / Organics
https://thrivemarket.com/food?utm_source=google&utm_medium=cpc&utm_campaign&Desktop-Generic&utm_content=16383675632&utm_term=%2Borganic%20%2Bfood%20coupons&device=c&gclid=CJ2H9Zux3skCFYeRHwodS88OAw

Door-to-Door Organics
https://tristate.doortodoororganics.com/signup?gift_cert=organics&gclid=CL33iZ6z3skCFccYHwodJ3oH2A

Try your local co-op, health food store, Whole Foods Market, Trader Joe, and most large grocery store chains for organics: meat, vegetable protein, vegetables, grains, seeds, fruits, and nuts.

GMOs: Genetically modified organisms called 'phood'

One of the most serious problems about eating unhealthfully, e.g., glyphosate-contaminated nutrition profiles, is the unavoidable and sordid reality that eaters don't know if—or what—they are eating has been genetically modified.

Since the latter part of the 1990s, GMOs have been making their way into mainstream food marketing and saturating markets without labeling, at the deliberate decree of the U.S. Food and Drug Administration (FDA), and much to the chagrin of numerous independent scientists who declare GMOs unsafe as human food[155].

Part of the reason is due to the fact that GMO crops are sprayed inordinately with the herbicide glyphosate, which has been declared a "probable carcinogen" by the International Agency for Research on

---

155 http://www.collective-evolution.com/2014/04/08/10-scientific-studies-proving-gmos-can-be-harmful-to-human-health/ accessed 3-5-16

Cancer (IARC) of the World Health Organization on 20 March 2015. This is what IARC said in a press release:

"The herbicide glyphosate and the insecticides malathion and diazinon were classified as probably carcinogenic to humans (Group 2A)."

The particular herbicide that must be used to grow GMO crops, by legal contracts farmers sign, is Roundup® manufactured by Monsanto. Glyphosate is the active ingredient in Roundup®. It's an endocrine disrupter that blocks and disrupts multiple metabolic pathways, e.g., aromatase activity and mRNA[156].

Furthermore, one of the most respected researchers of GMO science and information, the Institute for Responsible Technology—Jeffrey M Smith, claims that the GMO process creates massive collateral damage in GMO plants thereby causing mutations in hundreds, if not thousands, of locations throughout the plant's DNA, which humans and animals, in turn, eat as 'phood'.

The American Academy of Environmental Medicine (AAEM) released this statement to its physicians regarding GMOs:

"Physicians to educate their patients, the medical community, and the public to avoid GM (genetically modified) foods when possible and provide educational materials concerning GM foods and health risks. [....] Several animal studies indicate serious health risks associated with GM food..."

Those scientific studies confirm these health harms from GMOs to the study animals: infertility, immune problems, accelerated ageing, insulin regulation, and changes in major organs and the gastrointestinal tract.

---

156 http://www.gmfreecymru.org/pivotal_papers/crucial5.htm accessed 2-17-16

Coincidentally, since 1996 when GMOs were marketed, the rise in chronic diseases parallels the rise in the use of glyphosate. In 2015, over three hundred million pounds of glyphosate were sprayed on crops and soil.

Apparently, and according to a published report in 2010[157], researchers discovered that certain *Enterobacteriaceae* lead to Inflammatory Bowel Disease, Crohn's, and Ulcerative Colitis.

Additionally, according to Barling and Brooks, *"The genes of genetically modified foods are split with the E. coli bacteria, Bt toxin and other 'gene promotors' that leave the bacterium's residue in your gut that causes IBD, IBS, Crohn's and ulcerative colitis. It didn't get there by accident. The statistical increase in digestive diseases and colorectal cancer can be directly traced to the creation of genetically modified foods and the addition of dangerous addictive chemicals in packaged foods."*[158]

GMO crops are produced as: *Transgenic* (a foreign genetic element [DNA/RNA] inserted to confer a new trait) and *Cisgenic* (introduction of genotype changes rather than genetic engineering—no transgene) either to be herbicide tolerant and to be insect resistant.

To further 'enhance' GMOs pest infestation-defeating-capabilities, the herbicide glyphosate must be considered. It is the active ingredient in Roundup®, the primary Monsanto herbicide used on GMO crops labeled "Roundup Ready"[159], which have been patented to withstand and resist Roundup® spraying and applications, thereby leaving residues in and on growing crops.

---

157 http://www.cell.com/cell-host-microbe/fulltext/S1931-3128%2810%2900276-3 accessed 3-23-16
158 http://howtoeliminatepain.com/attention-crohn%e2%80%99s-and-ibd-sufferers-%e2%80%93-harvard-researchers-discover-the-obvious-about-how-genetically-modified-foods-lead-to-inflammatory-bowel-disease-crohn%e2%80%99s-and-ulcerative-c/ accessed 11-10-15
159 http://www.sourcewatch.org/index.php/Roundup_Ready_Crops accessed 11-17-15

One of the more important aspects of glyphosate is that it interferes with and destroys the shikimate pathway in plants sprayed, while also depleting the good bacteria in the agricultural ecosystem. Somehow, GMO science was able to buffalo federal approving agencies about the shikimate pathway, since humans don't have that pathway. However, glyphosate has tragic impacts upon the plants' shikimate pathway! Soil bacteria DO have a shikimate pathway, and humans have millions of good bacteria in our gut—the gut microbiome—which glyphosate drenched crops and foods wreak havoc with. Jeffrey Smith of the Institute for Responsible Technology and Dr Stephanie Seneff, PhD, (MIT research scientist) discuss the shikimate pathway and glyphosate/GMOs in an hour-long interview at http://wyebrookfarm.com/an-interview-with-jeffery-smith-and-dr-stephanie-seneff-glyphosate/.

Furthermore, glyphosate, an endocrine disruptor, has been dubbed a "hormone hacker"[160].

Probably, the ultimate shocker for readers will be to learn, especially if you favor imported German-made beer, that a substantial number of those beers have been tested for glyphosate residues and here are the findings:

Hasseroder Pils	*29,74 µg/l (ppb)*
Jever Pils	*23,04 µg/l*
Warsteiner Pils	*20,73 µg/l*
Radeberger Pilsner	*12,01 µg/l*
Veltins Pilsener	*5,78 µg/l*
Oettinger Pils	*3,86 µg/l*
Konig Pilsener	*3,35 µg/l*
Krombacher Pils	*2,99 µg/l*
Erdinger Weisbier	*2,92 µg/l*
Paulaner Weisbier	*0,66 µg/l*
Bitburger Pils	*0,55 µg/l*

---

160 http://detoxproject.org/glyphosate/hormone-hacking/ accessed 2-29-16

Beck's Pils   0,50 µg/l
Franziskaner Weisbier   0,49 µg/l
Augustiner Helles   0,46 µg/l
ppb = parts per billion
Resource: *Sustainable Pulse*, the Munich Environmental Institute[161]

Which foods are GMO engineered?

Alfalfa, which is cattle feed
Animal foods (cheese, dairy, eggs, meat, yogurt, ice cream, etc.) from GMO-fed, factory-farmed animals, rBGH injected cows
Apples (Arctic, a green apple which prevents browning)
Artificial additives, sweeteners and preservatives
Cassava (starchy root)
Cooking oils, especially Canola, Corn, Cottonseed, and Soy [My suggestion: use organic grapeseed oil, which has a high-burning temperature and plenty of antioxidants for high-heat cooking, if you must use high heat or fry foods]
Corn (90% of U.S. crop)
Cotton seeds are used to make cottonseed oil for food processing
Flax
Hawaiian Papaya
Honey in Canada due to GMO canola prevalence; in the USA, 75% of honey on grocery store shelves was found to contain high fructose corn syrup, which is a GMO product—90% of corn in USA!

---

161 http://sustainablepulse.com/2016/02/25/german-beer-industry-in-shock-over-probable-carcinogen-glyphosate-contamination/#.VtX462z2b9I accessed 2-29-16

Jatropha, which are the seeds of the Jatropha plant that is *used like palm oil* and for feeding livestock
Milk (rBGH growth hormone)
Peas
Plum
Potatoes: Innate® and approved Ranger Russet, Russet Burbank and Atlantic produced by J.R. Simplot
Rice, e.g., "Golden Rice"
Rose
Salmon (AquAdvantage brand salmon can be grown as farm raised)
Soy (95% U.S. crop)
Squash: Yellow and Zucchini
Sugar beets
Tobacco 90% of U.S. tobacco crop (Are smokers smoking glyphosate herbicide? What does that do to human lungs?)
Tomatoes
Yeast, e.g., GMO wine yeast ML01; bakers and beer yeasts

Another disconcertingly miserable, but true, fact regarding the herbicide glyphosate, which is used on GMO crops while growing, is that farmers began using glyphosate for pre-harvest crop staging as a drying and ripening agent just before harvesting non-GMO crops such as wheat, sugarcane, peas, beans, lentils, and many other crops which, undoubtedly, leaves toxic residues in/on those crops. Coincidentally, a study done on UK and Scottish wheat and barley[162] indicates that as much as 17 percent of breads sampled from 2000 to 2006 contained glyphosate residues! Can glyphosate be part of the gluten intolerance problem?

---

162 http://cereals.ahdb.org.uk/media/185527/is02-pre-harvest-glyphosate-application-to-wheat-and-barley.pdf_accessed 11-28-15

Additionally, 160 crops have been approved for glyphosate staging and spraying 3 to 5 days before crop harvests. Shouldn't that be a defining reason to eat organically-grown foods?

The other downside of glyphosate is a metabolite it produces in plants—aminomethylphosphonic acid (AMPA)[163], which is a little less toxic than glyphosate.[164]

In a 2014 issue of the *Journal of Organic Systems*[165], four researchers published the paper "Genetically engineered crops, glyphosate and the deterioration of health in the United States of America." It's a 32-pager that "talks turkey" about the apparent health effects from glyphosate—the main ingredient in Roundup®, which is sprayed copiously on GMO/GE crops growing in the fields, leaving residues in them.

That paper discusses correlation analyses regarding glyphosate, GMOs, GE corn, GE soy, and toxicology apparently impacting Alzheimer's disease, autism, bladder cancer, cancer, senile dementia, diabetes, hepatitis C, hypertension, inflammatory bowel disease, intestinal infections, kidney cancer, kidney failure, lipoprotein metabolism disorder, liver cancer, multiple sclerosis, myeloid leukemia, obesity, pancreatic cancer, Parkinson's disease, end stage renal disease, and thyroid cancer with alarming increase rates. Their research indicates that the last 20 years represents the same time period when there was an exponential increase in the use of glyphosate on food crops, especially GMOs or genetically engineered crops. They documented that there was a 527 million pound *increase* in herbicide use between 1996 and 2011.

---

163 http://jxb.oxfordjournals.org/content/early/2014/07/18/jxb.eru269.full accessed 11-28-15
164 http://www.ncbi.nlm.nih.gov/pubmed/21190714 accessed 11-28-15
165 http://www.organic-systems.org/journal/92/JOS_Volume-9_Number-2_Nov_2014-Swanson-et-al.pdf accessed 2-4-16

Their research also indicates a sudden increase in chronic diseases in the mid-1990s, which coincides with the commercial production of GMO crops.

Some reports are surfacing that Morgellons disease[166] also may be associated with genetically modified 'phoods'. However, I'm more inclined to think that weather geoengineering and spraying[167] of chemtrails as part of the government's Solar Radiation Management program are contributing to that very recent and exacerbating health problem.

Scientists are wondering what effects stacking two transgenic inserts into one GMO maize/corn hybrid may do to impact the overall expression of endogenous genes, especially protein changes and the "safety" of stacked transgenic crops. There's a 2014 published report about that, which can be found at the URL address http://bmcplantbiol.biomedcentral.com/articles/10.1186/s12870-014-0346-8. How does that geoengineering impact zein, a class of prolamine protein in corn and maize? Could corn also be causing gastrointestinal issues like wheat, even though corn is touted as "gluten free"?

Ironically, the U.S. EPA is considering putting limits on genetically engineered corn. The reason is because some of the pests GE corn was designed to defeat, well, those pests—the corn rootworm, in particular—have evolved to resist the genetically-engineered-bug-killing corn crop! To add insult to injury for GE seed companies, the corn rootworm is one of the most cost-expensive pests attacking the corn crop, and those little critters outwitted science!

It is imperative, from my perspective as a consumer health researcher for close to 40 years, author, retired practicing *natural* nutritionist, and

---

166 http://www.mayoclinic.org/morgellons-disease/art-20044996 accessed 11-17-15
167 http://www.geoengineeringwatch.org/ accessed 11-17-15

breast cancer survivor, that all food eaten in order to beat *any and all diseases* must be non-GMO and preferably verified as such on product labels. Foods should have the proper coding sticker on all fresh produce with the number "9" preceding the PLU (Price Look-Up) food number, e.g., organic bananas are coded 94011.

Theoretically, there are three numbers in the PLU code system for identifying fresh foods:

0 – Applies to non-qualified produce
8 – Applies to genetically modified produce (GMOs) but no one is using it, it seems!
9 – Applies to organic produce and it is used in the USA

Another helpful product-identification icon is the *Non-GMO Project* [168] label, which verifies there are no GMOs in the product. Check out that project on the Internet. However, some in the GMO-labeling movement think the best assurance is found in the USDA's organic label[169], which means it's not GMO or GE; products have been grown adhering to government standards for organics, i.e., 95 percent—no less than that—of the ingredients are organic and non-GMO; and animal-source foods (meat, milk/dairy products, eggs) contain no antibiotics or growth hormones.

In addition to the above, some food processors use what's called "reverse labeling" regarding GMOs whereby the producer indicates somewhere prominently on the label "No GMOs". Many canned food labels now also indicate "BPA-free can."

---

168 http://www.nongmoproject.org/product-verification/ accessed 2-18-16
169 https://www.organicconsumers.org/news/can-consumers-trust-usda-organic-label-food-products-china accessed 2-18-16

Any parent trying to find help for a child on the Autism Spectrum, or who may be vaccine damaged, needs to change the child's diet to a *totally GMO-free food plan* without exception, in my opinion, and that of holistic physicians working with, and even curing, ASD children. My suggestion is to research the work being done by Dr Zack Bush, MD, triple board certified, which I discuss at the end of this chapter and before the Resources.

There's another broad-spectrum herbicide—glufosinate—that's problematic insofar as it's sprayed as a pre-harvest chemical to facilitate even crop harvesting—as is Roundup®[170], in addition to GMO crops for weed control. Canola, corn, cotton, and soy beans are both GMO glufosinate- and glyphosate-resistant crops, which mean they are sprayed liberally with those herbicides for weed control and for staging harvests. If anything, that alone, ought to convince you to eat organically-grown food.

Finally, a film has been produced, which documents the journey Kathleen DiChiara and her family took to restore their health from many (21) chronic health disorders (allergies, asthma, auto-immune disease, autism—plus others). *Secret Ingredients* is a film worth watching because it will help you to understand the importance of eliminating GMOs, glyphosate, and pesticides from your food and diet, and how eating organically-grown and produced foods will restore your body to exceptional health.

The trailer for the film *Secret Ingredients* can be watched here https://www.youtube.com/watch?feature=player_detailpage&v=CnXG3-Vt2Ps#t=15.

---

170 http://roundup.ca/en/preharvest accessed 11-17-15

How to repair GMO-chemical damage to your body
Two websites:
http://easyhealthoptions.com/gmos-happens-lab-just-half-danger/
http://easyhealthoptions.com/ingredient-food-corporations-want-keep-hidden/ expounds upon information with renaming all GMO-'phoods' to date.

Recently, and while writing this book, I learned of *triple-board-certified* Dr Zack Bush, MD,[171-172] and his research work regarding *intestinal wall tight junction breaks* resulting from glyphosate residues found in food. Tight junctions, biologically speaking, are "fire walls" of protection, formed by the fusion of integral proteins in lateral cell membranes of adjacent epithelial cells thereby limiting trans-epithelial permeability, or what Dr Bush calls "a communication network disruption" among cells. Dr Bush is getting remarkable results with repairing those tight junction breaks. Besides diet, nutrition, and life style changes, Dr Bush uses *Restore*® supplement to promote gut microbiome repair and recolonization. Furthermore, he thinks gluten intolerance also results from tight junction breaks in the intestinal wall. The same also can happen at the blood brain barrier, which he offers is the cause of "brain fog."

Dr Bush's protocol restores the cellular communication network and disrupts the chronic inflammation cycle caused by glyphosate, which was patented as an "antibiotic" to deal with parasites in humans and animals[173-174].

---

171 https://www.youtube.com/watch?feature=player_detailpage&v=GzyLxuiUz0U#t=66 accessed 2-17-16
172 https://www.youtube.com/watch?feature=player_detailpage&v=pbNV7jM_poQ#t=65 accessed 2-17-16
173 http://www.google.com/patents/US7771736 accessed 2-17-16
174 https://gmoanswers.com/ask/why-did-monsanto-patent-glyphosate-antibiotic-also-medical-estab-

Resources

The Institute for Responsible Technology – Jeffrey M Smith
http://responsibletechnology.org/gmo-education/articles-about-health-risks-by-jeffrey/

EPA Used Monsanto's Research To Give Roundup A Pass
https://theintercept.com/2015/11/03/epa-used-monsanto-funded-research/

Jeffrey Smith, The Institute for Responsible Technology, interviews Dr Zack Bush, MD (Revolution Health Center) on how to repair the human gut after eating GMOs. (1 hr 7 min YouTube video)
https://www.youtube.com/watch?v=-S-daTpxImE&feature=player_embedded#t=78

"By the end of this call, I hope you realize that it is really the story of the gut lining and its loss of communication with the bacteria that is causing most global injury that we are suffering as a society now from the loss of bacterial diversity."

Food and Chemical Toxicology: Vol. 84, October 2015, Pg. 133-153
Potential toxic effects of glyphosate and its commercial formulations below regulatory limits
http://www.sciencedirect.com/science/article/pii/S027869151530034X

Dr Patrick Moore, an obvious GMO golden rice promoter, rejects drinking Roundup® when challenged to do so after he's remarked that you can drink a quart of it and it won't harm you! You have to see this one. https://www.youtube.com/watch?feature=player_detailpage&v=ovKw6YjqSfM#t=9

---

lishment-has-been-preaching accessed 2-17-16

Food Buying, Storing, and Preparation

---

*We spend good money, at times, for worthless foods.
The most important features of nutritious foods
are how they are grown, stored, and prepared.
This chapter, hopefully, can impart how important
food buying, storing, and preparation really are.*

Storing Certain Foods

The way your groceries are stored, after bringing them home, will have great impact not only on taste but with regard to nutritional values, too.

Fruit

For example, bananas are not digestible until many brown spots have covered the peel, which indicates that the starches have converted into digestible sugars. Never refrigerate bananas, as that hinders ripening and their peels turn black. However, ripe bananas can be peeled and placed in containers in the freezer in order to make frozen banana custard, if you have the correct food processing machine[175]. It is great

---

[175] http://www.thekitchn.com/how-to-make-creamy-ice-cream-with-just-one-ingredient-cooking-

tasting, too, and an excellent nutritional substitute for commercial ice cream. See the chapter, *Ice Cream That Can Be Nutritious Too*.

Another fruit, which actually is eaten and regarded as a vegetable, the tomato, should not be placed in the refrigerator. Allow tomatoes to mellow in sweetness, ripeness, and taste in an airy basket or dish at the far end of the kitchen counter, away from stove or toaster oven heat. Refrigeration retards tomatoes ripening and flavor, I feel. Here's a tomato hint: To cut any tomato perfectly, use a serrated knife or a bread knife. It's like magic with no squashed tomatoes!

I'm a firm believer in not refrigerating "stone or pit center fruit," e.g., apples, nectarines, peaches, pears, etc., but leaving them in a fruit basket on the kitchen counter so that the starches in them can turn into digestible sugars thereby making them sweeter and more digestible.

However, berries, cherries, grapes, melons, and pineapples—once cut, definitely need refrigeration.

Whole citrus fruits can stay in a fruit basket on the kitchen counter or in the refrigerator. Personally, I think room temperature foods have much more flavor than ice cold food—but that's my opinion.

There's nothing like a 'hand' of fresh organic ginger for adding zing to a recipe or making fresh ginger-lemon tea. Ginger can be stored on the kitchen counter for about a week or 'naked' in a refrigerator crisper—meaning, not in a plastic bag, which will cause moisture to form and get slimy.

Herbs

Herbs like fresh cilantro, dill, and parsley often are sprayed with so much water in stores to keep them fresh, that when you refrigerate them, they

---

lessons-from-the-kitchn-93414 accessed 12-24-15

turn slimy within a day or two. I constantly complain about all the fluoridated water that is sprayed on organically-grown food, but green grocers just can't seem to make the connection.

Consider chopping those freshly-purchased herbs and storing them in the freezer to spoon into recipes. Woody herbs like fresh thyme can be frozen whole on their branches and put into soups and stews that way. The leaves cook off and impart their wonderful flavors. Basil leaves, when very fresh, can be plucked off the plant stems and placed flat on to a cookie sheet and flash frozen in the freezer, then transfer them to a plastic container to use in soups, stews, and cooking other dishes. They taste like fresh basil. Frozen basil leaves, however, don't work in salads or other fresh recipes; they "melt."

If you can grow your own fresh windowsill or kitchen garden herbs, so much the better. I remember years of gardening with herbs and running out to quickly snip off some fresh chives, basil, sage, thyme, mints of all kinds while cooking, plus edible herb flowers to decorate my salads.

Even though fresh herbs are wonderful to use in cooking and as garnishes, they can become a problem because of their turning mushy or slimy very easily. That's why I like to purchase and use dried organically-grown herbs for most of my cooking. I find it less frustrating and definitely more cost effective with very little waste.

If I can find a *dry* bunch of parley, which I love to use as fresh garnish on many vegetable dishes, it can keep well in a breathable plastic bag in the refrigerator crisper for about a week before it starts to break down. In summer, I have a pot of Italian parsley growing on the back patio of my condo townhouse. However, the caterpillars love it too.

I prefer to leave heads or bulbs of garlic on the kitchen counter in a fruit basket unless, of course, you purchase the ready-to-use, peeled garlic, which needs to be refrigerated. I don't like that the 'paper' skin on garlic can get slimy, wet, and moldy in the refrigerator.

Vegetables
All fresh vegetables should be stored in the refrigerator crisper in breathable plastic bags and used or eaten with a few days of purchase for best nutritional values. I don't recommend storing salad greens in the bags in which they are purchased, as they turn yucky too easily. I transfer them to breathable plastic bags or recycled plastic tubs other greens, like baby spinach, come in.

Potatoes, sweet potatoes, yams, and onions all should be stored in a cool dry place in the kitchen. Potatoes should be kept in a dark area, e.g., a breathable container under a kitchen cabinet to avoid solanine (a plant toxin) forming due to exposure to light[176]. Green potatoes NEVER should be eaten, as you can get very sick from them.

Beans and Grains
Dry beans and grains, I suggest, should be removed from their packages once opened and transferred to glass jars with metal lids for safe keeping. The same for pastas, as no bugs or mice can get at them through the packaging. Furthermore, you readily can see what they are and how much you have on hand. Recycle glass jars as food containers instead of throwing them in the trash.

Canned Groceries
For any canned goods, e.g., soups, coconut milk, pumpkin, organic beans, etc., please remember to wash the lid and dry it carefully before opening it with a can opener, as there can be anything on it like

---

176 http://www.accessdata.fda.gov/scripts/plantox/detail.cfm?id=1364   accessed 12-24-15

chemical bug sprays from where it was stored, bug particles, dried vermin urine, dirt, etc. Also, remember to wash the can opener head and dry it to keep it clean and free from bacteria.

For any canned goods that you open in glass jars, like jams, jellies, nut butters, etc., I recommend washing the inside of the lid and drying it before placing it into the refrigerator. That little trick will prevent mold from growing quickly on the inside of the lid and contaminating the contents of the jar while in the refrigerator. I can't tell you how many cooks have thanked me for that hint.

Animal Source Foods

All animal source food products must be refrigerated. Make certain you check the cold-keeping-quality of the refrigerator with a refrig thermometer from time to time. Don't store eggs in a door shelf; place them on the back of a refrigerator rack to keep them cold. Make it a habit to clean the inside of the refrigerator often; keep an open container or ramekin dish of baking soda inside the refrigerator to maintain a fresh air quality.

Plastics in the Kitchen

I'd like to caution that most plastic wrap, freezer bags, sandwich bags, and baggies for food storage can be made with chemicals like polyvinyl chloride (PCV), phthalates, or bisphenol A (BPA). Know that there are kitchen plastics made without those toxic chemicals. One brand I know of and use is *Whole Foods 365 Everyday Value*. Also, I suggest wrapping cheeses in waxed paper first, then use plastic wrap. I also suggest using a paring knife to scrape off all sides of the cheese after you've taken it out of the store plastic and before placing it in your refrigerator. Better yet, use a small porcelain crock with a lid to store cheeses. Cheese will stay fresher longer, too.

Cooking Pots, Pans, and Utensils

I definitely recommend not using non-stick pots, pans, or fry pans since they are coated with toxic chemicals like Teflon. The Environmental Working Group maintains a "PFC Dictionary"[177] listing of perfluorinated and perfluorochemical coatings, which you ought to become familiar with, plus the reasons for not cooking with such toxic-like cookware[178]-[179].

Stainless steel[180], ceramic porcelain coated cast iron, and tempered glass (Pyrex, Corning) are what I would recommend. Definitely NO aluminum pots, pans, molds, cookie sheets, baking and pie pans, etc.[181] I'm not very happy with iron frying pans, as I think they may be problematic insofar as the possibility of transferring too much iron into foods or not being able to be kept as bacteria-free as they should be, especially due to the fat-based coating that needs to be built up to "cure" them. But that's my opinion.

I don't use silicone utensils either. I prefer real wood or stainless steel cooking utensils. The fewer man-made chemicals used to make kitchen utensils, the less likely a "chemical migration" or leaching during heat and pH transfer is possible, at least to my way of thinking.

Chopping boards can become problematic, I think. I don't recommend plastic since the cutting action and pH factors of food enzymes and juices can and may become involved with possible transfer into chopped foods. But that's my concern. I use solid wood chopping boards, which I do NOT oil, but wash with very warm water, dish soap,

---

177   http://www.ewg.org/search/site/teflon%20dictionary accessed 3-21-16
178   http://www.ewg.org/research/healthy-home-tips/tip-6-skip-non-stick-avoid-dangers-teflon accessed 3-21-16
179   http://www.ewg.org/key-issues/toxics/nonstick-chemicals accessed 3-21-16
180   http://butterbeliever.com/how-to-tell-quality-of-stainless-steel-cookware/ accessed 3-21-16
181   http://www.newsmax.com/Health/Health-News/cookware-dangers-teflon-alzheimer/2013/07/10/id/514282/ accessed 3-21-16

and use a scrubby or Bon Ami cleanser to clean off the board and rinse very well. My chopping boards are over 25 years old and look brand new, with the exception of knife marks, but no stains or discolorations.

Microwave Ovens
This probably will not sit very well, but I do not recommend microwave oven cooking or even reheating of cooked foods, *especially a baby's bottle!* Even the FDA does not recommend heating a baby's bottle in a microwave: *"Heating breast milk or infant formula in the microwave is not recommended. Studies have shown that microwaves heat baby's milk and food unevenly. This results in "hot spots" that can scald a baby's mouth and throat."*

Even though the FDA's reasons are different than mine, they still make sense. Furthermore, according to a Dr Mercola published article, *"Heating the bottle in a microwave can cause slight changes in the milk. In infant formulas, there may be a loss of some vitamins. In expressed breast milk, some protective properties may be destroyed."* [182] Dr Hans Hertel researched the effects of microwave cooking on food; that it changes the molecular structure of food; plus the effects of microwaved food on the body.[183]

There is one kind of radiation microwave ovens freely emit into the environment: thermal infrared radiation. This is because they are at room temperature, and all objects at room temperature emit thermal infrared radiation. (Scary note: Your microwave oven emits thermal infrared even when it's unplugged!) [184]

---

182 http://www.mercola.com/article/microwave/hazards2.htm accessed 3-21-16
183 http://www.globalhealingcenter.com/natural-health/why-you-should-never-microwave-your-food/ accessed 3-21-16
184 http://rationalwiki.org/wiki/Microwave_oven accessed 3-21-16

Did you know that the Russians banned microwave ovens in 1976, but that ban was lifted after *Perestroika* (1985-1991)? Russian forensic research teams studying microwave ovens and cooking produced this information:

- *Heating prepared meats in a microwave sufficiently for human consumption created:*
  - *d- Nitrosodiethanolamine (a well-known cancer-causing agent)*
  - *Destabilization of active protein biomolecular compounds*
  - *Creation of a binding effect to radioactivity in the atmosphere*
  - *Creation of cancer-causing agents within protein-hydrosylate* [hydrolysate] *compounds in milk and cereal grains;*
- *Microwave emissions also caused alteration in the catabolic (breakdown) behavior of glucoside - and galactoside - elements within frozen fruits when thawed in this way;*
- *Microwaves altered catabolic behavior of plant-alkaloids when raw, cooked or frozen vegetables were exposed for even very short periods;*
- *Cancer-causing free radicals were formed within certain trace-mineral molecular formations in plant substances, especially in raw root vegetables;*
- *Ingestion of micro-waved foods caused a higher percentage of cancerous cells in blood;*
- *Due to chemical alterations within food substances, malfunctions occurred in the lymphatic system, causing degeneration of the immune system=s* [sic] *capacity to protect itself against cancerous growth;*
- *The unstable catabolism of micro-waved foods altered their elemental food substances, leading to disorders in the digestive system;*
- *Those ingesting micro-waved foods showed a statistically higher incidence of stomach and intestinal cancers, plus a general degeneration of peripheral cellular tissues with a gradual breakdown of digestive and excretory system function;*
- *Microwave exposure caused significant decreases in the nutritional value of all foods studied, particularly:*

- *A decrease in the bioavailability of B-complex vitamins, vitamin C, vitamin E, essential minerals and lipotrophics* [fat breakdown]
- *Destruction of the nutritional value of nucleoproteins in meats*
- *Lowering of the metabolic activity of alkaloids, glucosides, galactosides* [monosaccharide sugar from lactose] *and nitrilosides* [B17] *(all basic plant substances in fruits and vegetables)*
- *Marked acceleration of structural disintegration in all foods.*[185]

Microwave Resource

Are Microwaves Compromising Our Health?
https://www.rethinkingcancer.org/resources/articles/are-microwaves-dangerous.php

Food Preparation

Preparing food is one of the greatest gifts a person or cook can give to others, I believe. I'm of the esoteric mindset that if you don't add love to your cooking, it lacks a key ingredient. Today's quick, fast food eating and lifestyle don't offer much in the way of interacting with food to enjoy it as we should, in my opinion. Eating on the run causes digestive problems, too.

Personally, I think families should sit down together every evening and enjoy a homemade meal together. Family members could help in preparing dinner, too. One member could do the salad; another prepares one or two vegetable side dishes; while Mom or Dad prepares the main course entrée. A volunteer can do the dessert, if one is needed. That way a sense of family cohesiveness and unity not only is enforced, but food becomes a focal and important part of family life. As it stands now, I'd guess not many families can say that.

---

185 http://www.aaimedicine.com/jaaim/apr06/hazards.php?printable accessed 3-21-16

Furthermore, such practices will provide a tradition about food that younger family members will want to carry on when they leave the nest. Food is a social feature in life. How many friends meet for lunch, dinner, or Sunday brunch?

Cleanliness

Cleanliness is paramount in food preparation. All foods should be washed before cooking to displace any untoward contaminants. Always check for dirt, bugs, etc. Beans and lentils should be picked over for hidden small stones. *Everything should be rinsed thoroughly before cooking.* Use a strainer colander as you clean and prep veggies.

Fresh fruits and vegetables, especially if not organically-grown, ought to be washed using a liquid fruit and vegetable wash that can remove pesticides, waxes, and chemicals. However, make certain the wash is not made with chemicals. One brand, *Environné*™, which I use, is made from plant oils, grapefruit seed, and lemon-orange extracts.

Keep hands washed while preparing food and have all cuts covered with a band aid or wear kitchen gloves. Don't put the same spoon you tasted the food with back into the cook pot without washing it or using a new, clean spoon. Hygiene is extremely important when preparing food, especially when making food for other eaters.

Salt

I'm a firm believer in NOT salting vegetable, grains, or beans cooking or soaking water. We eat too much salt in prepared and restaurant foods, so the best way to eliminate any salt overuse and/or craving is not to salt everything while cooking with the exception of making soups or other entrée dishes and then, use only a minimum of salt. Don't put salt into cooked cereal water either. Even though we need salt in our diets and bodies, we don't need all the chemicalized salts that we get in processed and restaurant-prepared foods.

High Heat Cooking

I think high heat cooking creates unhealthful ingredients in food, especially fried foods and starchy foods like potatoes (and chips), grain products (and chips), and coffee. French roast and Turkish coffee (espresso) don't get my vote either. They're roasted so that beans are burned dark, bitter, and taste that way, too, in my opinion. Besides the caffeine in coffee, can the intense, high-heat bean roasting give coffee "addicts" *agita,* a vernacular of the Italian description for heartburn: *"bruciore di stomaco agita?"* Acrylamides[186] probably are formed. What are acrylamides, you may be asking? According to the National Cancer Institute,

> *Researchers in Europe and the United States have found acrylamide in certain foods that were heated to a temperature above 120 degrees Celsius (248 degrees Fahrenheit), but not in foods prepared below this temperature (1). Potato chips and French fries were found to contain higher levels of acrylamide compared with other foods (2). The World Health Organization and the Food and Agriculture Organization of the United Nations stated that the levels of acrylamide in foods pose a "major concern" and that more research is needed to determine the risk of dietary acrylamide exposure.* [187]

That's why I'm a proponent of low heat cooking. You will find that my personal recipes instructions say to heat the pan or bring something to a boil, but turn down to medium or low heat. That's the reason, and more specifically, not to change the nutrition value and structure of cooking oil.

---

186 http://www.fda.gov/Food/FoodborneIllnessContaminants/ChemicalContaminants/ucm053569.htm#8 accessed 3-22-16
187 http://www.cancer.gov/about-cancer/causes-prevention/risk/diet/acrylamide-fact-sheet accessed 3-22-16

Other chemicals created by heat and cooking include PAHs—polycyclic aromatic hydrocarbons. We can be exposed to PAHs that occur in the environment[188], but we should not create them by cooking nutritious food incorrectly, I contend. How we cook meat, in particular, determines whether PAHs and/or heterocyclic amines (HCAs) are formed. According to the National Cancer Institute PAHs and HCAs have been found to be mutagenic, i.e., causes changes in DNA, which may increase our cancer risks, especially of the stomach and digestive tract, I offer.

When animal meats—and fats, in particular—are charred or touched by fire, PAHs and HCAs[189] are formed. Blackened and fire barbecued meats, chicken, or fish are first-rate ways of getting PAHs and HCAs from food, I offer.

Foods and Additives, Colors, Food Processing Chemicals, and Preservatives Once you realize how many chemicals are in food that you absolutely have no control over, you will become an avid label reader, I bet. Besides, one very distinctive piece of food information is not listed on food labels: genetically modified organisms—GMOs!

Reading labels is very easy to master. If you can't pronounce it or it's not a food crop like potato, rice, wheat, or animal product, but any one of hundreds, if not thousands, of food processing chemicals, which you can't recognize as real food, then the edibles in that package have been sullied with food processing chemicals, which you may not want to eat when you "eat to beat disease." Here's the FDA's "Food Additive Status List"[190], which you may want to print out and study. Plus there's

---

188 https://toxtown.nlm.nih.gov/text_version/chemicals.php?id=80 accessed 3-22-16
189 http://www.cancer.gov/about-cancer/causes-prevention/risk/diet/cooked-meats-fact-sheet accessed 3-22-16
190 http://www.fda.gov/Food/IngredientsPackagingLabeling/FoodAdditivesIngredients/ucm091048.htm accessed 3-22-16

something else to look out for: the "Color Additive Status List"[191] that you need to include, if you want to keep food coloring chemicals out of your body.

Something you may be interested in knowing is that not only is fluoride added to drinking water in many places, but fluoride also can be added to milk and salt in areas where municipal drinking water isn't fluoridated. According to a 2006 paper, "Legal aspects of fluoride in salt, particularly within the EU," by F. Gotzfried (*Schweiz Monatsschr Zahnmed* 116:371-75), the following countries fluoridated salt: Austria, France, Germany, Spain, and Switzerland. However, these countries fluoridate milk: Bulgaria, Chile, China, Peru, the Russian Federation, Thailand, and the UK (Britain). Since fluoride is a protoplasmic poison, you may want to find out if the salt and milk you purchase are fluoridated.

In my opinion as a retired healthcare professional and a thinking person, I cannot understand for the life of me how the U.S. FDA and USDA have allowed so much chemical contamination into foods we put into our bodies. That should be outlawed by law; not permitted by federal government agency regulations.

Happy food shopping!

---

191 http://www.fda.gov/ForIndustry/ColorAdditives/ColorAdditiveInventories/ucm106626.htm accessed 3-22-16

A Greasy Story about Cooking Oils

What would you think if I told you that I consider liquid cooking oil equivalent to cancer in a bottle? Shocking, you'd probably reply. Well, the more you learn about highly processed vegetable oils used in cooking, especially high heat and deep frying recipes, the more you may be inclined to agree with me, I think.

There are numerous types of oils with which to cook. Animal fats are eschewed as being "bad" fats, whereas highly processed and even chemicalized polyunsaturated plant-based oils are considered "good" fats. Nothing, in my opinion, is further from the nutritional facts, I offer. Another fat is even more dangerous health-wise – it's a synthetic fat, e.g., trans-fats, plus margarine, which is a manufactured substitute for butter, a real animal fat that human bodies have evolved with probably over several millennia.

Trans-fats and saturated plant-based fats are heated and treated exceptionally dangerously nutrition-wise, in my opinion. A process called hydrogenation is used to make both those fats. Liquid vegetable oil is heated with hydrogen atoms and a catalyst metal, e.g., nickel, palladium, or platinum, is added to the oil in order to make a liquid oil become a solid at room temperature.

Most cooking oils, which are classified as fats, start out as a plant-based crop from close to 25 fruits, seeds, and/or nuts. What you probably don't know is that herbicide toxins sprayed for pest control on any crop lodges in the fat-containing part of the crop, which is the seed or nut that is rendered into cooking oil. Many field crops, especially genetically modified ones like canola, corn, cottonseed, and soy, are sprayed with inordinate amounts of glyphosate and/or glufosinate herbicides, which, undoubtedly, leave residue in the fatty part of the plant. To make cooking oil, fruits, seeds, and nuts go through extraction and refinement processes, which add some interesting chemicals UNLESS the oil is produced by what's called the "cold pressed" process, as with extra virgin olive oil.

What's involved in extraction and refinement?
Extraction is done by expeller pressing whereby the oil can heat up to 120°F, which can lead to free radicals being formed in oil when it's exposed to heat. Then there's cold pressing during which the oil is not heated and results in nutritionally safer and healthier oil, in my opinion. There's chemical extraction in which the chemical hexane is used in extracting the oil from seeds like soy, peanuts, corn, and canola. As an FYI, *"rats, chronically exposed by inhalation to hexane, have exhibited neurotoxic effects."*[192]

Cooking oil refinement is another story altogether, and where the real nutritional nightmares begin, in my opinion. Here are the refinement processes that most cooking oils go through:

Distilling, degumming, neutralization during which the oils are treated with sodium hydroxide or sodium carbonate, bleaching

---
192 http://www3.epa.gov/airtoxics/hlthef/hexane.html accessed 11-20-15

and heating, dewaxing or winterizing, deodorizing and treating with high-heat pressurized steam—more heat equals more free radicals?, and preservatives like BHA and BHT are added *"to help preserve oils that have been made less stable due to high-temperature processing."*[193]

Two "food-preserving" chemicals unfortunately approved by the U.S. FDA – BHA and BHT – boggle my mind as to why they even are permitted to be used. According to Anne Marie Helmenstine, PhD,

"Both BHA and BHT have undergone the additive application and review process required by the US Food and Drug Administration. However, the same chemical properties which make BHA and BHT excellent preservatives may also be implicated in health effects. The oxidative characteristics and/or metabolites of BHA and BHT may contribute to carcinogenicity or tumorigenicity; however the same reactions may combat oxidative stress. There is evidence that certain persons may have difficulty metabolizing BHA and BHT, resulting in health and behavior changes."[194]

The last two sentences by Dr Helmenstine, I think, could corroborate my comment about cooking oil being equivalent to cancer in a bottle! What do you think?

Another equally, plus nutritionally questionable and relatively recent "in-vogue" food production oil is *palm kernel*, an inexpensive trans-fat replacement that's responsible for dramatic rain forest destruction due to deforestation creating palm tree orchards for oil production. Statistically, 80 percent of palm oil, if not modified, naturally is saturated fat—the bad fat for your heart! That being said, *palm fruit*

---

[193] https://en.wikipedia.org/wiki/Cooking_oil#Olive_oil_extraction.23Modern_method:_decanter_centrifugation accessed 11-20-15
[194] http://chemistry.about.com/od/foodcookingchemistry/a/bha-bht-preservatives.htm accessed 11-20-15

oil is very rich in vitamin E and lower in saturated fat. Some research indicates that palm kernel oil, which is high in palmitic acid, could be an inducement to eating more food and weight gain.

In 2005 the *American Journal of Clinical Nutrition* published a study (C Lawrence Klein, et al)[195] wherein an increase in palmitic acid, which is high in palm kernel oil, led to lower fat oxidation rates, plus a decrease in metabolism. The end result, according to that research, was a diet high in palmitic acid probably can increase the chances for obesity, including insulin resistance (diabetes?). Many pastries and munchies, especially those made by "health food" brands, use palm oil. Do your research and if you have digestive problems or bowel issues, check out the oils in your diet.

Now here's something to consider seriously: Research indicates that palm oil, due to its processing, is more difficult to digest.

Having given you documented information about cooking oils, I must tell you that the only oil I use in my cooking is organically-grown, Extra Virgin Olive Oil—preferably from Italy or Spain—which means the very first pressing with all the nutritional values still remaining in the oil. Olive oil, however, can be processed and refined several ways, e.g., Extra Virgin, Virgin, Pure, and Light olive oils. I recommend only Extra Virgin Olive Oil and endorse using it with low heat cooking.

Coconut oil currently is being touted as very healthy oil. Personally, I stay away from it, as it's a naturally occurring high-saturated fat! The fat in coconut oil is 92 percent saturated fat! The LDL content in coconut oil is not very healthful for your heart. According to the Pritikin Longevity Center, *"Ounce for ounce, coconut oil has more saturated fat than butter, beef tallow, or lard."*[196] Did you know that?

---

195 http://ajcn.nutrition.org/content/82/2/320.full accessed 11-21-15
196 https://www.pritikin.com/your-health/healthy-living/eating-right/1790-is-coconut-oil-bad-for-you.html accessed 11-20-15

The saturated fat in butter is 65 percent, compared to coconut oil, which is 92 percent saturated fat! *In my opinion,* grass-fed, pasture-raised butter is a much healthier fat than any of the commercially processed vegetable oils except cold pressed, extra virgin olive oil.

Regardless of the nutritional spin and sales pitches put out about various cooking oils, for maximum health benefits *you must consider particular non-advertisement issues*: whether the source product (crop, seed, nut, fruit) is genetically modified; if it's been grown organically without herbicides; and most importantly, how it's been processed into free flowing oil—something that does not exist naturally in Nature. Fat/oil always comes encased within fiber or tissue because Nature knows that's how it can be digested properly. Heating oil—especially using high-heat, e.g., deep frying—in my opinion, ought to be considered the "mortal sin" of cooking. Once you evaluate how you feel after eating cooking oils and fats, you will begin to realize what you must do to attain wellness regarding cooking oils and fats in your diet.

The only cooking oil I use and recommend since my studies in the 1970s and '80s is extra virgin olive oil. However, it's not used commercially very much because it's a more costly-to-produce product: cold pressed rather than expeller or chemically-extruded vegetable oils, which promote inflammation and disease in the body, as far as I'm concerned. Furthermore, highly-touted polyunsaturated vegetable oils are nutritionally dangerous[197].

Most polyunsaturated oils are used because they are touted as being able to withstand higher cooking heat and frying. In my opinion, no foods should be deep fried and eaten! Heating oil causes chemical changes in the oil. In November of 2015, *The Telegraph*, a London online newspaper, published "Cooking with vegetable oils releases toxic

---

197 http://paleoleap.com/many-dangers-of-excess-pufa-consumption/ accessed 1-21-16

cancer-causing chemicals, say experts"[198], which I encourage everyone to read online. It will open your eyes not only how to eat, but how to cook, thus explaining why all my recipes use E.V. olive oil and medium low heat to cook.

Another article I refer you to is "Mediterranean diet plus olive oil may reduce breast cancer risk"[199] published online by Reuters, which I encourage everyone to read.

For salad dressing, make your own using E.V. olive oil! Or, do as I do: Dress a salad with freshly squeezed lemon juice and E.V. olive oil drizzled on. Sprinkle some dried herbs: dill weed, basil, and oregano, along with Himalayan pink salt and cayenne pepper. Voilà—instant Italian dressing! By the way, bottled salad dressings probably are not good for your health, in my opinion. Read their ingredient labels, plus highly processed polyunsaturated oils.

Since this chapter discusses only cooking oils—not essential fatty acids (EFAs) per se—I'd like to caution you that your diet should be structured to obtain adequate EFAs daily. A plant-based diet that is well researched and followed, which includes "eating a rainbow of foods," i.e., many colored fruits and vegetables, legumes, nuts, and seeds, will give you a proper balance of Omega-3 EFAs to Omega-6 EFAs, which is most important for everyone's overall health and well-being. EFAs are discussed in the chapter, *EFAs: The fats you really need—Essential Fatty Acids*.

However, there may be a possible tasteless side to extra virgin olive oil, which you should be aware of and factor in when purchasing olive oil. Late in 2015, Italian prosecutors investigated the allegations that

---

[198] http://www.telegraph.co.uk/news/health/news/11981884/Cooking-with-vegetable-oils-releases-toxic-cancer-causing-chemicals-say-experts.html accessed 1-21-16
[199] http://www.reuters.com/article/us-health-oliveoil-breast-cancer-idUSKCN0RE25B20150914 accessed 1-21-16

several of the top extra virgin olive oil exporters (Antica Badia, Bertolli, Carapelli, Coricelli, Primadonna, Santa Sabina, and Sasso) allegedly cut their extra virgin olive oil with lesser quality oils!

Tests apparently confirmed that nine out of every 20 bottles of oil tested that were produced by those exporters were tainted with other oil(s) and not strictly pure extra virgin olive oil. It seems that canola and soy bean oils were imported and mixed into and sold as extra virgin olive oil. That means GMOs were most likely included in the olive oil, since canola and soy are high GMO crops in the USA and Canada. However, the companies involved in the "olive oil adulterations" cite false testing procedures.

But, what you ought to know is that for restaurants there's an "olive oil" blend produced called "Virginola"™[200], which is a mixture of extra virgin olive oil blended with canola or soy oils, that restaurants pawn off as cooking with "olive oil". Be aware if you either are allergic to canola or soy, or if you don't want to eat GMO oils. Some restaurants claim they use olive oil but instead may be using a blended olive oil.

My suggestion is to ask the wait staff at a restaurant claiming to cook with olive oil to check with the kitchen or chef to ascertain if their olive oil is 100% pure olive oil or a blended olive oil like Virginola™.

Better still, to make certain you are buying what you want and are paying for, cold-pressed, preferably organically-grown, extra virgin olive oil, make certain that it smells and tastes like raw olives! Many boutique food shops offer tastings, which I love to sample. My late husband and I treated olive oil like many collectors treat wine. We loved the varieties of olive oil from around the Mediterranean area. Currently, I'm using a lovely organically-grown, extra virgin olive oil from Morocco.

---

[200] http://www.trademarkia.com/virginola-all-natural-blend-85119011.html accessed 1-21-16

Healthful dietary oil is important to attaining and maintaining vibrant health. Your skin will not age; your endocrine system will function as Nature programmed; your intestinal tract will not be compromised, since oils and fats affect the ecological balance of the bowel.

Once you've attained wellness again, a variety of organically-grown foods can be added in moderation, including sustainably-grown animal products in moderation, if you so choose. However, I do not recommend changing cooking oils; extra virgin olive oil is the cooking oil of choice for good health, in my opinion.

Resources to check out online

Trans-fats are double trouble for your heart health
http://www.mayoclinic.org/diseases-conditions/high-blood-cholesterol/in-depth/trans-fat/art-20046114 accessed 11-20-15

Why Hydrogenated Oils Should Be Avoided at All Costs
http://www.naturalnews.com/024694_oil_food_oils.html   accessed 11-20-15

Big fat truth about cooking oil and cancer
http://easyhealthoptions.com/big-fat-truth-cooking-oil-cancer/   accessed 1-21-16

EFAs: The fats you really need—Essential Fatty Acids

The low-fat craze, in my opinion, is nothing short of crazy! Why? Because the body absolutely needs certain fats, either from animal, but especially from plant sources, to be healthy. No ifs, ands or buts about it, in my opinion. The body uses fat to manufacture tissue and hormones, plus "oil your joints"[201], colloquially speaking. However, I eschew canola oil and don't recommend it—period!

The fats we are familiar with in our bodies are triglycerides, cholesterol, and fatty acids. However, we even have *visceral fat* around vital abdominal organs to protect them. Did you know that? There's a right amount of visceral fat to protect organs and then there's a wrong amount—the type that protrudes out and makes men look like they are nine months pregnant. That is very troublesome visceral fat and needs to be downsized in order to avoid diseases like type 2 diabetes, heart disease, and cancer. Such a physique usually results from too many starchy carbs, fatty red meats, and trans- fats, I offer. Oh, don't forget the beers, too. Carbs, carbs, and more carbs, which turn into fat!

---

201 http://www.arthritis.org/living-with-arthritis/arthritis-diet/best-foods-for-arthritis/healthy-oils.php accessed 3-16-16

Fat in the diet does not mean you necessarily will have an obese body. As matter of fact, in order to lose weight, your diet should have the correct amount of proper fats![202] *There should be some correct fat eaten with every meal,* e.g., fatty fish like salmon, cholesterol in an egg, monounsaturated oil like extra virgin olive oil, or avocado, olives, walnuts/nuts, and seeds.

Why should we eat some fat with our meals? First, fat not only provides satiety, but it helps with digestive processes and provides essential fatty acids—those healthy fats our bodies can't manufacture but need for optimum health. Those important EFAs are Omega-3 and Omega-6. Then there's Omega-9, a less important, *and sometimes troublesome*, fat, I contend. Most EFAs can be obtained from plant-based sources.

Omega-3 EFAs

These fats cannot be manufactured by the human body. There are three main Omega-3s:

> *Eicosapentaenoic acid* (EPA) and *docosahexaenoic acid* (DHA), which are found in fish—salmon, halibut, sardines, anchovies
>
> *Alpha-linolenic acid* (ALA) found in vegetable oils and nuts (especially walnuts), flax seeds and *high lignan* flaxseed oil that should not be used for cooking but as a supplement, leafy vegetables, and *some animal fat, especially grass-fed animals*[203]

Omega-6 EFAs

The body cannot manufacture these EFAs, which are contained in:

---

202 http://www.fitnessmagazine.com/recipes/healthy-eating/tips/why-non-fat-isnt-the-answer/ accessed 3-16-16
203 http://www.grassfedgirl.com/omega-3-foods/ accessed 3-16-16

Avocado, *whole grains* and cooked whole grain cereals, eggs, nuts, poultry, most vegetable oils, and some meats, e.g., pork

One important thing to keep in mind about Omega-6s is that they can be *pro-inflammatory* and *anti-inflammatory*, depending upon individual body chemistry metabolism and one's constitution, which most food advisers don't take into consideration, in my opinion, or even mention: individual biochemistry. One-size nutrition does not fit everyone. Nutritional needs and sources depend upon on how YOUR body metabolizes food and interacts with its internal and external environments, I offer.

Omega-9

Not many people are familiar with Omega-9 fatty acids, since technically it's not classified as an EFA, since the body can manufacture it. Omega 9s are monounsaturated fats—while 3s and 6s are mostly polyunsaturated fats—found in food. There are two Omega-9 acids that are "exploited" by industry: Oleic acid and Erucic acid. Erucic acid can cause gastrointestinal distress. Because it was so predominant in rape seed oil, the sale of rape seed oil was prohibited in the USA by the FDA.

> *"Erucic acid was enough of a concern that in 1956, the U.S. Food and Drug Administration (FDA) banned rapeseed oil for human consumption. In addition, demand for rapeseed meal was low because of high levels of glucosinolates, a compound that at high doses depresses animal growth rates."* [204]

Erucic acid is found in rapeseed, wallflower seed, and mustard seed.

---

[204] http://www.ers.usda.gov/topics/crops/soybeans-oil-crops/canola.aspx accessed 3-16-16

But here's where genetic engineering and modification came into play by Canadian food scientists in the 1960s and rape seed morphed into canola:

"Rapeseed with high erucic acid content is grown for commercial use in paintings and coatings as a drying oil. Canola oil comes from a cultivar of the rapeseed plant that has been bred, or in some cases genetically modified, to contain very little erucic acid." [205]

Folks with gastrointestinal problems, I offer, cannot tolerate even the smallest amount of erucic acid that's been left in altered/GM canola oil. I think it may have something to do with "leaky gut" syndrome, plus the ratio of Omega-6 being out of balance with Omega-3. There can be some side effects to consuming canola oil[206] that both the health food industry [tsk, tsk, tsk] and food processors in general, including restaurateurs, either overlook or deliberately use in wanting to keep production costs lower even though there is risk of canola negatively impacting the microbiome, *in my opinion,* for people with gluten intolerance, leaky gut, irritable bowel syndrome, etc.

Canola oil, in my opinion, ought to be considered detrimentally-equivalent to gluten for those who can't handle it. However, it's in everything – or almost everything!

An Israeli study published in the November 1996 issue of the *Israeli Journal of Medical Sciences* concluded, *"Thus, rather than being beneficial, high omega-6 PUFA diets may have some long-term side effects, within the cluster of hyperinsulinemia, atherosclerosis and tumorigenesis* [tumor-causing]*."*[207]

---

205   https://en.wikipedia.org/wiki/Omega-9_fatty_acid accessed 3-16-16
206   http://www.livestrong.com/article/153341-canola-oil-side-effects/ accessed 3-16-16
207   http://europepmc.org/abstract/MED/8960090 accessed 3-16-16

Canola oil is a relatively high Omega-6 PUFA—polyunsaturated fatty acid—20 percent by ratio.

Now, I'd like to share with you what I wrote about EFAs in my 2012 book, *A Cancer Answer,* since fats play an important role in defeating cancer:

Why are these fats so important in our daily diets? Research and published papers reveal they:

- Affect many inflammatory responses and cellular activity.
- Provide cellular signaling.
- Activate and inhibit DNA transcription factors.
- Affect our mood and behavior. Low dietary Omega-3 fatty acids are linked with depression.

Most cooking oils are polyunsaturated or monounsaturated (olive oil). Keep in mind that the optimum healthful ratio of Omega-6 (n-6) to Omega-3 (n-3) should be more Omega-3 n-3 than Omega 6 n-6, or a ratio range of one-to-one to one-to-four (1:1 to 1:4).

Here are the ratios of Omega-6 (n-6) to Omega-3 (n-3) for the more popular cooking and vegetable oils:
Canola: 2 (n-6) to 1 (n-3)
Furthermore, most canola is genetically modified to withstand glyphosate pesticide [herbicide], which is sprayed in inordinate amounts on GMO-canola.

Corn: 46 (n-6) to 1 (n-3)
Most corn is *bt*-corn, genetically modified to grow its own herbicide *Bacillus Thuringiensis.*

Cottonseed: just about none to none
Most cotton crops are genetically modified *bt*-cotton that grows its own herbicide *Bacillus Thuringiensis*.

Olive: 13 (n-6) to 1 (n-3)

Soybeans: 7 (n-6) to 1 (n-3)
Most soybeans (87-90% in USA) are genetically modified to withstand glyphosate pesticide [herbicide], which is sprayed in inordinate amounts on GMO-soy.

Peanuts: almost none to none

Another way of looking at the ratio of Omega-6 to Omega-3 is to *consider the percentages of those fatty acids in various oils:* Canola 20% (n-6) to 9% (n-3); Corn 54% (n-6) to 0% (n-3); Cottonseed 50% (n-6) to 0% (n-3); Soybean 51% (n-6) to 7% (n-3); Peanut 32% (n-6) to 0% (n-3); Flaxseed oil [organic] 14% (n-6) to 57% (n-3).

Never use flaxseed oil in cooking. Heat negates Omega-3 fatty acids.[208]

According to the University of Maryland Medical Center:

"A healthy diet should consist of roughly 2 – 4 times fewer omega-6 fatty acids than omega-3 fatty acids. The typical American diet, however, tends to contain 14 – 25 time more omega-6 fatty acids than omega-3 fatty acids."[209]

---
208 http://www.amazon.com/Cancer-Answer-Management-Effective-Treatments/dp/1477490175 Pp. 262-263 accessed 3-16-16
209 http://umm.edu/health/medical/altmed/supplement/flaxseed-oil accessed 3-16-16

Furthermore, the above research also indicates, *"Many researchers believe this* [ratio] *is a significant factor in the rising rate of inflammatory disorders in the United States."* [210]

The most important thing I think you need to know about EFAs is always make certain of the type of cooking oil you are using and eating, plus having a respectable amount of healthful fats in your daily diet. High lignan organic flaxseed oil fits the bill, in my opinion. You can use flaxseed oil as a salad oil and dressing.

The USA Institute of Medicine actually has not established a Daily Value (DV) for Omega-9 fatty acids. For amounts recommended for Omega-3 and Omega-6 EFAs, perhaps a safe, organic nutritional supplement ought to be investigated to make certain you are getting sufficient essential fatty acids, which your body cannot manufacture, especially if you eat a vegan diet, i.e., no animal products.

EFAs are so involved in body chemistry that I've not begun to even touch the surface. That would require a book all to itself. However, what I've shared with you, I feel, is the nitty-gritty about essential fatty acids, which seems not to be common knowledge.

Resources to check out
Book: *Fats That Heal, Fats That Kill: The Complete Guide to Fats, Oils, Cholesterol and Human Health* / Udo Erasmus / 1993 / Amazon.com

Book: *Eat Fat, Get Thin: Why the Fat We Eat Is the Key to Sustained Weight Loss and Vibrant Health*/ Mark Hyman, MD / February 2016 / Amazon.com

---

210 Ibid.

Food Families and Allergies

During my practice as a consulting *natural* nutritionist, I made it an emphatic point of reference for clients to know, or find out, if they were allergic to other foods they were not aware of. They possibly could have been allergic to other foods of a same "food family" to which a known offending food belonged. Here's an example: Say you are allergic to apples, then there's a probable likelihood that you also could be allergic to pears and quince, which are in the same food family.

That food family-allergy-relationship is something most eaters aren't aware of. It's almost like being allergic to your cousin, in some ways. However, the more important singular difference with food families is that, unknowingly, your immune system may, and can, be compromised if you are not aware of the potential harm for what could be termed "hidden food allergies," while regularly eating foods that are compromising your immune system.

Any food allergies—known or hidden—play overarching roles in body chemistry, which can result not only in digestive problems, urticaria (hives), even a more serious reaction—anaphylaxis, but more often than not, in contributing to chronic disease and inflammation within the body, which also can program, and result in, serious weight gain problems[211]. Compounding that is the fact that, according to the U.S. Centers for Disease Control and Prevention (CDC) estimates, 2 percent of adults and between 4 to 8 percent of children in the USA have food allergies. If you would like to know more about food allergens, may I suggest your checking out the November 2015 "FSIS Compliance Guidelines Allergens and Ingredients of Public Health Concerns: Identification, Prevention and Control, and Declaration Through Labeling" online[212].

Personally, I disagree with that report's statement on page 5 wherein it says,

Consumption of some ingredients, such as sulfur-based preservatives (sulfites), lactose, FD&C Yellow 5 (Tartrazine), gluten, and monosodium glutamate (MSG), may result in an adverse reaction in certain susceptible individuals, yet they are not considered allergens.

Man-made chemicals in food, water, and the environment absolutely induce and/or cause allergic responses, but government health agencies won't recognized that, I think, because all of allopathic medicine is built upon pharmaceutical drugs, which are legal chemicals dispensed as medicines. Pharmaceutical reactions are called "Adverse Reactions" rather than allergic reactions. To know more about drug reactions, I suggest accessing online "Worst Pills, Best Pills"[213].

In my practice, when I would meet with a client for the first time, I would make a special note to document if there was body puffiness, especially affecting the lower leg muscles. I came to realize that what appeared to look like "turkey drumsticks" could be associated with "body

---

211 http://www.food-allergy.org/inflammation.html   accessed 11-15-15
212 http://www.fsis.usda.gov/wps/wcm/connect/f9cbb0e9-6b4d-4132-ae27-53e0b52e840e/Allergens-Ingredients.pdf?MOD=AJPERES   accessed 11-17-15
213 http://www.worstpills.org/public/page.cfm?op_id=4   accessed 11-17-15

language" indicating some allergic responses to hidden food allergies in individuals. That tell-tale "body language" always prompted me to ask about and even delve into food allergies and/or to suggest the client keep a daily food diary to determine if he/she noticed any differences after eating, e.g., tiredness, itching, indigestion or excess flatulence, rapid pulse, perspiration, etc., and to log such corresponding information alongside a food or meal. Those foods then would be placed on a rotational diet, i.e., every 4 days or only once a week, to ascertain if there were "hidden" allergic reactions. One almost "fool proof" indicator associated with hidden food allergies is foods eaten daily or very often, plus irresistible cravings.

Why is it important to know if we are allergic to any foods, especially those we crave?

To rid the body of disease, it must be functioning at maximum efficiency on "all cylinders." If not, you will not obtain the desired results—health, plus you probably will be self-intoxicating the body instead of supplying maximum nutritional input. Furthermore, inflammatory diseases like Crohn's disease and Irritable Bowel Syndrome (IBS) usually become chronic. Leaky gut is the most prevalent problem stemming from or even causing food allergies, usually associated with gluten intolerance, plus other offenders, including GMO 'phoods' and glyphosate residues, in my opinion.

Healing leaky gut entails removing offenders; providing maximum nutrition and fiber content; eating prebiotic foods to recolonize the gut microbiome; and supplementing with mega doses of probiotics, which should be done under the supervision of a medical doctor or health practitioner who can provide proper testing and/or guidance. I'd like to steer you to the chapter *GMOs: Genetically modified organisms called 'phood'* wherein I discuss the work of Dr Zack Bush, MD, in healing glyphosate-damage to the microbiome.

In order to "eat to beat disease," it is imperative that you cooperate with your body's digestive, assimilation, and elimination processes in order to eliminate all stress, strain, and inflammation while simultaneously attaining maximum physiological benefits.

Below is a listing of many of the most common foods eaten in the modern agricultural countries and their plant food "cousins."

Plant Family	Plant Food "Cousins"
Apple	apple (cider, vinegar), crabapple, pear, quince, quince seed
Banana	banana, plantain
Beech	beechnut, chestnut, chinquapin
Birch	filbert, hazelnut, wintergreen
Buckwheat	buckwheat, rhubarb, sorrel
Caffeine	heterocyclic compounds known as purines (alkaloid)
Anacardiaceae	cashew, mango, pistachio
Citrus	citron, grapefruit, kumquat, lemon, lime, orange, tangelo, tangerine
Cola nut	chocolate (cocoa), cola (kola) nut
Fungi	mushroom, truffle, yeast (baker's, brewer's, distiller's)
Ginger	Cardamom, East Indian arrowroot, turmeric
Goosefoot	beet, lamb's quarters, spinach, Swiss chard
Gourd (melon)	cantaloupe (muskmelon), casaba (winter muskmelon), Chinese watermelon, citron melon, cucumber, gherkin, honeydew melon, Persian melon, pumpkin, summer squash, watermelon, winter squash
Grape	champagne, grape, raisin, vinegar (wine), wine (grape)

Grass (Cereals)	bamboo, barley, corn (maize), hominy, malt (germinated grain), millet, oat, popcorn, rice, rye, sorghum, sugar cane, wheat (bran, germ, gliadin, globulin, glutenin, leucosin, proteose, whole)
Heath	black huckleberry, blueberry, cranberry, wintergreen
Laurel	avocado, bay leaf, cinnamon, sassafras
Fagaceae (Legythis)	Brazil nut
Lily	aloe, asparagus, chives, garlic, leek, onion, sarsaparilla, shallot
Mallow	cottonseed, marshmallow, okra (gumbo)
Mint	balm, basil, catnip, horehound, Japanese artichoke, lavender, marjoram, mint, oregano, peppermint, rosemary, sage, savory, spearmint, thyme
Morning glory	sweet potato, yam
Mulberry	breadfruit, breadnut, fig, hops
Mustard	broccoli, Brussel sprouts, cabbage, cauliflower, collards, garden cress, horseradish, kale, kohlrabi, mustard, radish, rutabaga, turnip, watercress
Myrtle	allspice, cloves, guava, myrtle, pimento
Nightshade	bell pepper, cayenne pepper, chili (paprika) (red pepper), eggplant, ground cherry, melon peat, potato (white), tobacco, tomato
Nutmeg	mace, nutmeg
Olive	jasmine, olive
Orchid	vanilla
Palm	cabbage palm, coconut, date
Papaya	papain, papaya

Parsley	anise, caraway, carrot, celeriac, celery, coriander, dill, fennel, parsley, parsnip
Pea (Legume)	acacia, alfalfa, black-eyed pea (cowpea), broad bean (fava bean), carob bean (St. John's bread), chick pea (garbanzo), common bean (kidney, navy, pinto, string or green), Jack bean, lentil, licorice, lima bean, mesquite, pea, peanut, soybean, tamarind, tragacanth gum
Pepper	black pepper
Pine	juniper, pine nut (Pignolia)
Pineapple	pineapple
Plum	almond, apricot, cherry, peach, nectarine, plum, prune
Poppy	poppy seed
Rose	black raspberry, blackberry, boysenberry, dewberry, loganberry, red raspberry, strawberry
Rubiaceae	coffee
Saxifrage	currant, gooseberry
Sunflower	absinthe (Artemisia, sagebrush, wormwood), artichoke, chamomile, chicory, dandelion, endive, escarole, Jerusalem artichoke, lettuce, oyster plant (salsify), safflower, sunflower seed, tansy, tarragon
Tea (Camellia sinensis)	tea (black, green)
Walnut	black walnut, butternut, English walnut, hickory nut, pecan

Herbs—culinary and medicinal—are not classified in "families" other than botanical genus and species, but they are placed into several categories:

1. Aromatic herbs
2. Astringent herbs
3. Bitter herbs
4. Mucilaginous herbs
5. Nutritive Food Stuffs
6. Stimulant herbs
7. Laxative herbs
8. Diuretic herbs
9. Saponin herbs
10. Alkaloid herbs

Generally speaking, culinary (cooking) herbs are not problematic, but in the event you are allergic to any, please refrain from using them in your food and beverages, including those that can be ingredients in liquors and cordials.

Medicinal herbs should be studied carefully and discussed with your healthcare practitioner before embarking upon a regimen, especially if you are taking allopathic prescription medication or undergoing chemotherapy and/or radiation, as some herbs may alter an Rx's potency.

A classic example of how food and prescription drugs can interact is grapefruit juice[214].

Online, there's a "Drug Interaction Checker" which can be accessed at http://www.drugs.com/drug_interactions.html.

---

214 https://en.wikipedia.org/wiki/Grapefruit%E2%80%93drug_interactions accessed 11-15-15

Foods High in Antioxidants

Antioxidants can prevent, and even reverse, cellular damage done by pro-oxidants and oxidation.
During oxidation, naturally-occurring body chemicals are altered and become free radicals, which damage DNA and parts of cells. The following foods are high in antioxidants:

Artichoke, Black bean, Black plum, Blackberry, Blueberry (wild & cultivated), Cranberry, Gala apple, Granny Smith apple, Grapes: red, purple, blue, Nuts, Pecan, Pinto bean, Plum, Prune, Raspberry, Red Delicious apple, Red Kidney bean, Red bean (small), Russet potato, Sweet cherry

Naturally-occurring *Antioxidants* and the foods in which they are plentiful:

- Allium Sulphur compounds: Garlic, leeks, onions
- Anthocyanins: Berries, eggplant, grapes
- Beta carotene: Apricots, carrots, mangoes, parsley, pumpkin, spinach
- Catechins: Red wine, tea
- Copper: Legumes, nuts
- Cryptoxanthins: Mangoes, pumpkin, red peppers

- Flavonoids: Apples, citrus fruits, green tea, onion, red wine, tea
- Indoles: Cruciferous vegetables such as broccoli, cabbage, cauliflower
- Lignans: Bran, flax seeds, Sesame seeds, vegetables, whole grains
- Lutein: Corn, leafy greens (such as collard greens, kale, spinach)
- Lycopene: Pink grapefruit, tomatoes, watermelon
- Polyphenols: Oregano, thyme
- Selenium: Whole grains
- Vitamin C: Berries, broccoli, kiwi fruit, mangoes, oranges, peppers, spinach
- Vitamin E: Avocados, nuts, seeds, vegetable oils, whole grains
- Zinc: Nuts

Many herbs and spices are very good sources of antioxidants too! They include Jamaican allspice, cinnamon, cloves, ginger, marjoram, oregano, dried red peppers (Pepperoncini), pumpkin pie spice mix, rosemary, sage, turmeric, and thyme.

They also contain anti-inflammatory properties to reduce inflammation, a precursor to numerous chronic diseases, including cancer. There are several foods that have what's considered the "best" antioxidant properties. They include blueberries, fermented vegetables, garlic, leafy greens, and Shiitake mushrooms.

Inflammation usually is a precursor to contracting some form of chronic disease. It's the natural physiological response of the body's tissues to harmful stimuli, e.g., infections, pathogens, damaged cells, or irritants, including toxic chemicals found in vaccines and prescription drugs[215], plus what's forced into us through food, water, and environmental factors, e.g., Solar Radiation Management, aka "chemtrails".

---

215 http://www.cdc.gov/nchs/data/factsheets/factsheet_drug_poisoning.htm   accessed 3-9-16

A diet that is built around a daily intake of foods high in antioxidants acts as an excellent prophylactic for warding off inflammation.

Beans: That wonderful "musical" fruit

Did you know there are 40,000 bean varieties worldwide? Also, that beans are a powerhouse of nutrition, especially plant proteins that, literally, can cost only a few pennies per serving? Talk about bang for your protein buck!

Beans are thought to have originated in South America, Peru in particular. Their popularity apparently was spread around the globe after Spanish explorers took them back during their New World explorations in the late fifteenth century. However, pulses—ancient beans—have been documented in biblical times. There's a story in the Old Testament about two brothers, Jacob and Esau, and their involvement with a bowl of lentil stew.

*And Jacob sod pottage: and Esau came
from the field, and he was faint:
And Esau said to Jacob, Feed me, I pray thee,
with that same red pottage; for I am faint:
therefore was his name called Edom. And Jacob
said, Sell me this day thy birthright.
And Esau said, Behold, I am at the point to die: and
what profit shall this birthright do to me? And Jacob said,
Swear to me this day; and he sware unto him: and he sold*

> *his birthright unto Jacob. Then Jacob gave Esau bread and pottage of lentiles; and he did eat and drink, and rose up, and went his way: thus Esau despised his birthright.*
>
> ... Genesis 25:29-34 King James Version, Public Domain

That must have been some lentil stew! But, that's what the ancients thrived on—pulses.

Nutritionally, beans and pulses are wonderful cholesterol-reducing foods due to their rich source of B vitamins and fiber, which also prevents blood sugar levels from rising too quickly. Beans, or legumes as they sometimes are called, also are good for the heart. There's an old adage about beans, which kids thought funny, that goes something like this:

> Beans, beans are good for the heart; the more you eat, the more you fart!

Beans also healthfully impact the microbiome of the gut, an important aspect of the human immune system. However, if you experience flatulence (farting) after eating beans, that may be indicative that there may not be enough digestive enzymes being produced by your pancreas, since two starches in beans—raffinose and stachyose—may not be digested easily by some folks.

The bean starch problem can be corrected very easily by the manner in which beans are cooked; pre-cook rinsing until no bubbling appears; the combinations of foods beans are eaten with—e.g., no fatty meats—pork and beans, for example; and by improving the gut microbiome with dietary enzymes and/or probiotic supplements. Macrobiotic cooks like to include a two-inch piece of dried Kombu seaweed in the bean cook pot to prevent bean music.

Beans and pulses most often are purchased either as dry staples, which take hours of soaking and cooking time, or as pre-cooked, canned beans, which, frankly, I prefer to use since they save lots of time and have almost the same nutritional value of soaked beans, *if you don't rinse canned beans.* However, one has to be certain the canned beans you purchase are: 1) organically grown; 2) packed in BPA-free cans or packages; and 3) are certified to be GMO-free.

There also are fresh beans such as Lima or Butter beans, Green beans—aka string, runner, snap or French beans, and Fava beans, which are very large broad, flat beans favored in Mediterranean cuisine. All three bean varieties can be purchased frozen or canned.

Lentils similarly are classified as legumes, just like beans. There are several types: Brown, green, and red. Brown lentils probably are the most commonly known and used for soups, stews, and veggie burgers. Green lentils—aka French lentils, which are my favorite, are used to make salads, but I use them for every type of lentil recipe since they seem to have a better flavor, according to my taste buds. Red lentils traditionally are used to make Indian dal and curry recipes, and for thickening soups.

A cup of cooked lentils will provide 90 percent of folate (B9—folic acid) DRI/DVs; 37 percent iron; 36 percent protein; and 63 percent fiber, plus other minerals and nutrients. There's an added benefit to eating lentils: They are natural chelators, which remove toxins from the body due to their high sulfur content.

Beans, peas, and lentils, classified as legumes, are the edible portion (seeds) of pods and technically are known as *Leguminosae.*

Statistically, eating beans and lentils twice a week—or more—is associated with a 24 percent less chance of contracting breast cancer. However, as a breast cancer survivor, I heartily recommend eating beans as often as possible. Sometimes I eat beans twice a day, depending upon what's left over in the refrigerator, e.g., hummus (chick pea spread), bean salad, or a cooked bean entrée that I reheat for lunch or dinner.

Once your taste buds get used to the exquisitely delicious taste and texture of beans and lentils, I'm certain you will enjoy them as much as I do. You can be assured that when you combine beans and lentils correctly to make a complementary protein, you will not be lacking in quality plant-based protein.

Complementary Protein Cooking
Because legumes do not contain the full spectrum of amino acids to make a complete protein like animal foods, cooks have to combine specific plant-based, amino-acid foods to create a total amino acid chain of proteins known as "complementary proteins."

However, dry beans contain between 21 and 25 percent plant protein by weight. Black or turtle beans are considered the most nutritious of the beans probably due to three anthocyanin flavonoids in their black skin: delphinidin, petunidin, and malvidin. Two other flavonoids, kaempferol and quercetin, nicely round out the black bean's flavonoid profile.

In order to make complementary proteins correctly, cooks should combine:

1. Legumes with grains, nuts, seeds, or dairy
2. Grains with dairy
3. Seeds with legumes

One of the ditties I used to teach my nutrition clients and cooking class students about food combing went like this:

Peas and rice are very nice; they don't jack up the grocery price.

Peas are legumes and rice is grain, which fulfills the number 1 combination above.

Personally, I like to add seeds (chia, flax, pumpkin—the only alkaline-ash seed, sesame, and sunflower) to green salads for added vegetable protein and a crunchy texture, instead of croutons especially for those who are gluten-intolerant. One of my favorite seed combinations is sprinkling toasted sesame seeds and Himalayan pink salt over a serving of hot, cooked brown rice eaten with homemade vegetable soup, which is my all-time favorite breakfast or brunch. I sprinkle chia seeds as a garnish on cut up fruit salad and pumpkin custard pudding (recipe in *Recipes from Catherine's Kitchen*).

Besides the taste and gelatinous consistency of chia seeds (a no-cook pudding recipe is in the *Sweet Treats* section of *Recipes from Catherine's Kitchen*), here are the nutritional values that ought to be a real "turn on" to eating them.

Chia seeds are a powerhouse of nutrition.
They have 2.5 times more plant based protein than kidney beans
3 times more the antioxidant power of blueberries
3 times more iron than spinach
6 times more calcium than milk
7 times more vitamin C than oranges
8 times more omega-3 fatty acids than salmon (5 grams of omega-3s)
10 times more fiber than brown rice
And 15 times more magnesium than broccoli

Who would have thought that such a tiny seed would hold such a nutritional profile?

Besides, 2 tablespoons, or 1 ounce, of chia seeds contain 139 calories, 4 grams of plant protein, 9 grams of fat, 12 grams of carbohydrates, 11 grams of fiber, and antioxidants like Quercetin, Chlorogenic Acid, and Caffeic Acid, which actually prevent the seeds turning rancid. However, I always refrigerate chia seeds, as I do all seeds and nuts. They have fats in them, which can go rancid and become toxic, *pro-oxidants* with free radicals—the same thing can happen with oil fried seeds and nuts too. We should strive to eat as many anti-oxidants, rather than pro-oxidants, which deep fried foods become, in our diets as possible.

Once you introduce a variety of legumes and seeds into your diet, I think you will wonder what took you so long to realize just how delicious and nutritious they truly are.

Some of My Recipes for Beans and Legumes

Chick Peas Marsala
1 can Amy's Tomato Bisque soup [non-GMO, organic, dairy ingredient]
½ sweet onion, medium dice
¼ tsp Graham Marsala (Indian spice)
¼ tsp Himalayan pink salt
Pinch or two of cayenne pepper
1/8 tsp ground cardamom

Combine all ingredients into a small soup pot and bring to a boil; turn down heat/fire to medium low and simmer for 15 minutes.

Add
15 oz. can organic garbanzo (chick peas) beans, drained—don't rinse
Zest of 1 organic lemon rind
Cook for 30 minutes on low with a lid on the pot

Add
2 Tbsp. organic coconut milk-light and mix well
Cook on low for 10 minutes

Serving suggestion:

- Serve over cooked organic Basmati, Brown, or Wild Rice with a large green salad and steamed leafy greens, e.g., baby spinach, kale, Bok Choy, or broccoli.

Mung Bean Sauté (Gluten-free)

The day before soak overnight (24 hours), ½ cup dried mung beans in 2 cups of water. After several hours, pour off water, rinse well, and add fresh soaking water to cover the beans by 2 inches for the remainder of the soaking period. Keep beans covered. After 24 hours of soaking, mung beans are very tender and will cook in no time in the sauté recipe. Drain mung beans to use.

2 Tbsp. EV olive oil
¼ onion, minced
1 rib celery, minced
1 garlic clove, minced
10 button mushrooms, quartered
2 tsp fresh ginger, peeled and minced
1 Tbsp. Braggs Amino Acids (1 tsp more can be added, if needed)
½ tsp toasted sesame oil
Handful of fresh baby spinach leaves

Into a 10 inch stainless steel fry pan or wok, heat the oil; add onion, celery, garlic, mushrooms, and ginger. Mix well on medium heat for about 3 to 5 minutes
Add Braggs Amino Acids, mung beans, sesame oil, and spinach

On medium low heat, mix often for another 3 to 5 minutes until spinach is wilted and all ingredients are incorporated

Variation on the above recipe:
Instead of spinach, add a small handful of snow peas sliced into strips.

Mung Beans in Sauce Served over Grain
¼ cup mung beans soaked for 24 hours (overnight) and then they cook up in minutes.

2 Tbsp. EV olive oil
1 cup green cabbage, thinly sliced
¼ cup onion, chopped
3 Shiitake mushrooms, stems removed and sliced into thin strips
½ cup fresh fennel, thinly sliced from the bulb end
2 Tbsp. Braggs Amino Acids
1 tsp garbanzo bean miso mixed very well in ½ cup of water to make a smooth paste

Heat oil in a stainless steel fry pan, add veggies; turn heat to medium until veggies start to sweat
Add mung beans and Braggs Amino Acids
Cook 3 minutes, mixing often
Add miso paste, mix thoroughly to coat everything and cook for 1 minute on low heat.

Serving suggestions:

- Over cooked brown rice (gluten-free)
- Over cooked millet-and-brown-rice (Lotus Foods brand) ramen noodles (gluten free and a favorite presentation with guests)
- Over cooked barley (gluten)
- Over cooked quinoa (complete protein grain) (gluten-free)

Balance out the meal with

- A green salad
- Steamed asparagus
- Steamed broccoli

Christmas Lima Beans
These beans must be soaked a minimum of overnight, as they are large, beautifully colored beans.
Rinse well before cooking.

½ cup Christmas lima beans soaked and drained equals about 2+ cups beans after soaking
3 celery ribs, minced
1 sweet onion, minced
1 inch wide and long, organic lemon rind/zest
3 to 4 fronds of fresh thyme
¼ tsp Himalayan pink salt
Pinch or two of cayenne pepper
6 cardamom seeds ground in a mortar and pestle
Slight sprinkle of Chili Powder
3 cups water (a little more may be needed the longer beans cook)

Into a soup pot with a lid, combine all ingredients. Bring to a boil, turn down to medium low and cook with lid on for 2 hours. Mix often to keep from sticking to the pot, and make certain there is enough water.

Serving suggestion:

- These delicious beans make a wonderful entrée instead of meat.

Mixed Bean Chili

½ sweet red pepper, chopped medium
1 celery rib, chopped
1 large ripe tomato, chopped
½ sweet onion, chopped
1 tsp fresh ginger, peeled and finely grated
¼ tsp Himalayan pink salt
¼ tsp Chili Powder
Pinch or two of cayenne pepper
15 oz. can Westbrae Organic Salad Beans

Place all ingredients except Salad Beans into a 10 inch fry pan or skillet; add enough water to cover
Bring to a boil; turn down heat/fire to medium and cook for 3 minutes
Add 15 oz. can Westbrae Natural Organic Salad Beans, not drained
Cook on medium heat/fire for 15 minutes until thick

Serving suggestions:

- Serve as an entrée with a large tossed salad and cooked green vegetable, e.g., steamed asparagus or broccoli.
- Use as the filling for warmed-up organic tortilla shells topped with chopped lettuce, onions, and avocado, plus grated organic sharp cheddar cheese, if you eat dairy.
- Serve over a base of cooked quinoa with a huge mixed green salad and a side of steamed kale dressed with fresh lemon juice, EV olive oil, salt and pepper.

Lentil Salad

½ cup organic French lentils picked over, rinsed, cooked until tender, cooled and fluffed as you would rice
½ cup organic couscous (wheat pearls) or millet (grain) cooked until tender, cooled and fluffed

1 small carrot, small dice
1 rib of celery, small dice
8 cherry tomatoes, quartered
¼ red onion, chopped finely
Fresh lemon juice: ½ to 1 lemon juice, depending upon your taste for lemon
2 Tbsp. organic extra virgin olive oil
¼ tsp Himalayan pink salt or to taste
Pinch or two of cayenne pepper
½ to ¾ tsp dry tarragon herb (depending upon your taste)

Into a serving bowl combine lentils, grain, carrot, celery, tomato, onion. Set aside.
Prepare dressing by combining in a separate bowl: lemon juice, olive oil, salt, cayenne pepper, and tarragon leaves. Mix well. You can use a hand-held infusion blender to blend the dressing.

Pour dressing over lentils and veggies; mix very well. Refrigerate for at least an hour before serving.

Serving suggestions:

- Side vegetable dish or as an entrée
- Serve as appetizer on crackers, rice cakes or crackers, or toast points
- Filling for a wrap with shredded lettuce and/or sprouts, sliced tomato, and avocado

Sautéed French Lentils (Gluten-free)
1 cup cooked French lentils or 1 15 oz. can organic lentils drained, not rinsed
½ cup inner yellow stalks of celery, minced
½ sweet onion, minced
½ carrot, shredded
½ tsp dried tarragon leaves

¼ tsp Himalayan pink salt
Pinch or two of cayenne pepper
2 Tbsp. olive oil

In a 10 inch stainless steel fry pan, heat the oil; add celery, onion, and carrot
Cook on medium heat until onion is transparent
Add lentils, tarragon, salt, and pepper
Cook on medium heat until lentils are heated through, less than 5 minutes. If mixture gets too dry and starts to stick, add 1/8 cup water (or a few tablespoons of lentil can water) and mix well.
Don't overcook!

Serving suggestions:

- This dish can be eaten hot or as a cold salad atop mixed salad greens with cherry tomatoes, cucumber slices, and radish coins.
- Use as an entrée served with green mixed salad and two or three steamed vegetables.

Spicy Lentils (Gluten-free)
½ cup lentils picked over and rinsed very well
2 cloves garlic, chopped
½ sweet onion, diced
½ tsp grated fresh ginger
¼ tsp Himalayan pink salt
¼ tsp ground turmeric
Light sprinkling of Korintje cinnamon
½ tsp honey (mild)
2 cups water

Combine all ingredients into a pot with a lid. Bring to a boil and turn heat/fire down to medium low. Cook with lid on pot for about 45 minutes until lentils are soft and tender. Mix often to keep from sticking to the pot. A little water may be needed to keep the liquid from cooking away.

Serving suggestion:

- Make Spicy Lentils your entrée and round out the meal with a mixed green salad with cucumbers, radishes, sweet red pepper, lemon juice, olive oil and topped with sprinkling of dried basil, dill and oregano, plus steamed broccoli, steamed asparagus, and a side of fermented red beets.

Minted Garbanzo Bean and Cucumber Salad (Gluten-free)
1 15 oz. can organic garbanzo (chick peas) drained, not rinsed
½ cup English cucumber, skin on if organic, chopped
10 grape tomatoes cut in half
¼ cup red onion, minced

Dressing
Juice of 1 lemon with 2 Tbsp. of water added
3 Tbsp. extra virgin olive oil
1 clove garlic put through a garlic press (optional)
¼ tsp Himalayan pink salt
Pinch or two of cayenne pepper
½ tsp dried mint leaves

Into a serving bowl, combine garbanzo beans, cucumber, tomatoes, onion. Set aside.

Into a small bowl, combine lemon juice with water, olive oil, garlic, salt, pepper, and mint leaves.
Mix very well using a hand-held infusion mixer. The dressing will become a little thick as everything gets very well emulsified.
Pour dressing over veggies and mix very well.
Refrigerate an hour before serving.

Serving suggestion:

- Side vegetable dish
- Serve over greens as a salad course
- Great after-school or anytime snack

Scrambled Tofu—Not Eggs—for Breakfast (Soy—Gluten-free)
¼ lb. firm tofu, mashed (one-fourth of a tub of tofu)
¼ tsp turmeric
1/8 tsp curry powder
2 Tbsp. water
2 Tbsp. EV olive oil
2 mushrooms, small dice
¼ cup onion, small dice OR 3 scallions, chopped
¼ cup sweet red pepper, small dice
Optional: parsley chopped for garnish

Prep tofu first
Mash tofu in a small bowl using a fork; add turmeric, curry powder, and water.
Mash and mix until everything is thoroughly incorporated. Set aside.

Scramble tofu
Heat oil in a stainless steel fry pan; add mushrooms, onions, peppers.

Sauté veggies for 3 minutes on medium heat and mix constantly so veggies don't stick or brown.
Add prepped tofu and place a teaspoonful of water into the tofu bowl to rinse out the bottom and add it to the fry pan.
Scramble on medium low heat for about 2 to 3 minutes.
Serve as you would serve regular scrambled eggs. Garnish with chopped parsley.

Tofu Cacciatore (Soy)
2 Tbsp. EV olive oil
1 cup onion, chopped
1 cup sweet red pepper, julienned
1 heaping cup Cremini or Baby Bella mushrooms sliced medium thick
½ cup whole canned tomatoes, chopped, with juice
½ cup organic white wine (Sauvignon Blanc)
2 Tbsp. organic tomato paste mixed with 1 Tbsp. water
3 garlic cloves, chopped
¼ tsp turmeric
1 tsp honey
1 tsp dried basil
½ lb. firm tofu, cut into medium size cubes
Garnish: fresh parsley, chopped

Note: cook in an uncovered pot in order to allow wine alcohol to cook off/evaporate leaving only the taste.
Heat olive oil in a medium size soup pot
Add onion, red pepper, and mushrooms; cook, stirring often, until veggies sweat—about 3 - 4 minutes
Add tomatoes, wine, tomato paste, garlic, turmeric, honey, basil; cook 15 minutes on medium heat uncovered to create sauce

Add tofu and cook 5 minutes on medium low heat
Plate and garnish with chopped parsley.

Serving suggestion:

- As a bed for the cacciatore, serve cooked red quinoa, which I think is tastier than white
- Large mixed greens salad with some thinly sliced fresh fennel and thin sweet or red onion rings
- Steamed kale dressed with mashed avocado-lemon dressing
   Dressing Recipe: Combine ½ ripe avocado very finely mashed; juice of ½ lemon along with Himalaya pink salt and cayenne pepper to taste. This makes a paste-like dressing that, when added to hot steamed kale, thins out to coat the kale, adding a wonderful taste.

Mushroom Tofu Stir Fry (Soy)
2 Tbsp. EV olive oil
2 cups mushrooms, sliced
½ onion, chopped small
Pinch or two of cayenne pepper
2 Tbsp. Braggs Amino Acids
1 cup firm tofu, cut into small cubes
½ tsp toasted sesame oil
Garnish: chopped parsley and scallions

Heat olive oil in a 10 inch stainless steel fry pan
Add onion and mushrooms, mixing constantly for 4 minutes on medium heat
Add pepper, Braggs Amino Acids, and tofu; cook on medium low heat for 3-4 minutes
Remove from heat; add sesame oil and mix well to incorporate
Garnish with parsley and scallions

Serving suggestion:

- Bed of cooked millet-and-brown-rice (Lotus Foods brand) ramen noodles (gluten-free)
- Steamed veggie medley: broccoli, carrot coins, cauliflower, snow peas (done in a vegetable steamer that's inserted into a pot) drink the liquid that's left over—lots of nutrients there!
- Side of Kimchi—fermented Korean cabbage condiment

A Special Quick-fix Lentil Treat

This recipe cooks in less than 6 minutes since sprouted lentils, which have more nutrition due to sprouting, are used. The brand I use is *truRoots Accents Sprouted Lentil Trio.* There are green, brown, and black lentils that cook up very fast and very tasty, I think, using my following recipe. I like to eat left overs cold!

1 cup water
1/3 cup sprouted lentil trio
1 tsp Braggs Amino Acids
¼ tsp dried tarragon

Bring water to a boil in a pot with a lid; add lentils, Braggs, and tarragon. Reduce heat to simmer for 4 minutes with lid on the pot.
Remove from heat and let stand with lid on pot for 2 minutes.
Drain lentils or remove them using a slotted spoon, as the broth left over is delicious and can be used to add to veggies or to the following recipe.

After the sprouted lentils are cooked as above, sauté chopped onions and chopped mushrooms in some EV olive oil until they sweat; add drained lentils. You may need a little of the lentil cook water to keep it moist. Cook 2 minutes to incorporate everything. Delish!

Grains: What's to eat besides wheat?

Every culture expresses its love affair with wheat by using countless menu offerings, whether it is pita bread, matzo, croissants, spätzle, pasta, naan, donuts, or numerous variations of breads and rolls. Although wheat was referred to as the "staff of life," today it's just about been demonized for what the protein in wheat—gluten—does inside the human gut: causes discomfort and pain! We now have gluten-free memes just about everywhere. So, what other grains are there?

Grains are categorized as gluten and non-gluten.

Grains with gluten

For individuals who aren't bothered by leaky gut, or are not gluten-intolerant, there's barley, rye, spelt, teff, triticale, and wheat (durum, einkorn, emmer, farro, kamut, semolina—with each having individual protein earmarks), which I contend should be organically grown and not subject to herbicide staging pre-harvest.

Wheat is the prime ingredient in countless products, e.g., biscuits, bulgur, bread, cakes, cereals and cereal bars, couscous, crackers, crisp breads, crumpets, puffed wheat, Seitan, wheat bran and germ. Don't forget that wheat is used to make alcoholic beverages, too: American, Irish, and Scottish whiskey; some vodka is made from gluten-containing rye and barley; premium gins use wheat, rye, and barley; and beer is made from wheat. However, there's a gluten-free beer made from sorghum—"Redbridge" brand, a lager style beer, made by Anheuser-Busch.

The problem, nutritionally as I assess it regarding wheat, is that the more nutritious parts, bran and germ, are not used in making most commercial products, unless they are sold as whole wheat or whole grain. Most wheat products use only the starchy white endosperm, which is white flour, usually bromated[216].

Unless wheat or other grains are organically grown, there's the greatest likelihood that they go through a "staging" process several days before harvest when the crop is sprayed with the herbicide glyphosate[217]. That staging process also can be used on other crops too! They are: feed barley, tame oats, canola, flax, peas, lentils, soy beans, and dry beans[218]. Isn't that another verifiable reason to eat organically-grown food?

Personally, as a retired consulting *natural* nutritionist, I question whether it's the proteins in wheat, which humans obviously have eaten for eons of time, or is there some adverse gastrointestinal interactions between glyphosate and other herbicide residues in wheat; fumigants, if wheat was stored in grain silos; plus bromated wheat flour contains potassium bromate to improve the action of gluten during production.

---

216 http://www.ewg.org/research/potassium-bromate accessed 3-17-16
217 http://www.naturalnews.com/050583_glyphosate_wheat_bread_crop_contamination.html accessed 3-17-16
218 http://roundup.ca/_uploads/documents/MON-Preharvest%20Staging%20Guide.pdf accessed 3-17-16

Incidentally, the World Health Organization's IARC, has labeled potassium bromate a category 2B carcinogen—probable human carcinogen[219]!

So much for wheat! Incidentally, the Paleo diet discourages the consumption of cereal grains. I don't, but I do recommend that all grains be used with discretion, since the SAD diet is steeped in denatured grains and products: chips, crackers, donuts, pasta dishes, pretzels, and white bread—all of which turn into sugar during the digestive process and causes weight gain, fat accumulation, and messes with blood sugar metabolism.

Personally, I do not recommend a pour-out-of-the-box cereal for breakfast! If it's not a hot cooked, whole grain cereal, then it's a high carb starch, in my opinion. Hot whole grains like steel cut oats, Muesli, or quinoa topped with chia seeds and/or nuts with some Korintje cinnamon sprinkled on top, plus a teaspoon of honey mixed in, do not need dairy or nut milk. Toast or donut and coffee are not breakfast, I offer. That, in my opinion, is a bad snack to start your day. Breakfast is the most important meal of the day; it should be totally nutritious[220] to set up your body's metabolic system[221] for the day ahead after a nighttime fast while you slept.

Non-gluten Grains
Amaranth, buckwheat, brown and wild rice, cornmeal, millet, oats, quinoa, sorghum, and Montina—Indian Rice Grass flour that is super high in nutrition and protein, plus it tastes similar to wheat. Non-gluten grains are superb sources of nutrition. Almost all can be ground into flour.

---

219 http://monographs.iarc.fr/ENG/Monographs/vol73/mono73-22.pdf, Pg. 12 accessed 3-17-16
220 http://www.wholeliving.com/155850/healthy-breakfasts?tab=index accessed 3-18-16
221 http://www.responsiblefoods.org/how_does_the_metabolic_system_work accessed 3-18-16

In order to keep this book a manageable size for the reader, in this section on non-gluten grains, I will refer you to online websites where you can find numerous recipes for grains you probably never even thought about. *One thing I want to suggest is always to use organic, non-GMO ingredients, and you can substitute ingredients, e.g., if a recipe calls for margarine, substitute pasture-raised butter or a safe oil. Use aluminum-free baking powder—Rumford is a brand. For recipes that contain a lot of sugar, I'd just forget about them until you learn how to substitute honey or other natural sweeteners in baking.*

Amaranth

Dr Andrew Weil, MD, has a great recipe[222] for making amaranth for breakfast and also popping it like one pops corn. I'm directing you to his website so that you can learn more about amaranth and realize that there are medical doctors who know something about nutrition. Furthermore, Dr Weil was a member of the Medical Advisory Board of the national coalition I was Executive Director for five years in the 1980s. He's one of the "pioneering MDs" in the holistic approach to health.

Buckwheat

This website[223] has twenty recipes using buckwheat, e.g., buckwheat apple ring cake; buckwheat pancakes—but I'd leave off the bacon, unless you eat meat and cook nitrate-free bacon from sustainably raised hogs; buckwheat granola; buckwheat biscuits; buckwheat risotto; buckwheat garden salad, plus others that should give you an idea of how to cook with buckwheat.

Brown and Wild Rice

Regarding rice, I have to caution you that arsenic has been found in some imported rice. Personally, I think the brand that is safe is

---

222 http://www.drweil.com/drw/u/ART03177/How-to-Cook-Amaranth.html accessed 3-18-16
223 http://www.huffingtonpost.com/2015/03/23/buckwheat-recipes_n_3795721.html accessed 3-18-16

Lundberg[224], grown in California, USA. Their website is complete with information about various types of rice and when you click on Recipes, you get a wealth of recipes for appetizers, breakfast, dessert, entrées, soups, and sides. Enjoy! Lundberg is the rice I cook with too.

Cornmeal

Again, I must mention that most of the corn crop in the USA is GMO, so purchasing and cooking with corn, including corn oil, corn starch, popcorn, chips, etc., should be from organically grown corn—blue, yellow, or white. *Cook's Illustrated* offers some interesting cornmeal recipes[225] like muffins, pancakes, spoon bread, and polenta.

Millet

I have to caution you about millet. I love it! Once you try it, you will find yourself in love with it too, I think. Millet has such a pleasant, clean, filling taste that goes with everything, and it doesn't take very long to cook. Here's a great recipe for millet cakes[226] that I think you will enjoy time and again.

This website features millet for breakfast with recipes[227] for pancakes, porridge, casserole, and smoothies!

Oats

Even though oats are considered gluten-free, they have another protein—*avenin*, which can cause an immune response and gut reaction in some folks, including those with celiac disease. So, be careful to make certain that if you think oats don't agree with you, cross them off your gluten-free list of grains.

---

224 http://www.lundberg.com/product/organic-brown-basmati-and-wild/ accessed 3-18-16
225 https://www.cooksillustrated.com/taste_tests/53-cornmeal accessed 3-18-16
226 http://www.loveandlemons.com/millet-cakes-carrots-spinach/ accessed 3-18-16
227 http://healthyeating.sfgate.com/eat-millet-breakfast-5272.html accessed 3-18-16

Dr Andrew Weil, MD, has a most informative webpage about oats that I think you ought to know about too, especially the four types of oats he thinks we should focus on eating.[228]

Quinoa

This ancient South American-native grain, called "the mother grain," comes in three varieties: black, red, and white. I must admit, red is my favorite. I eat quinoa for breakfast sometimes; as a bed for any vegetable entrée dish or saucy dish; as an extra tablespoonful added to a bowl of soup; or as a bed for a loosely scrambled egg in herb [229]butter and/or olive oil, topped with sprouts and scallion rings. Somehow that dish reminds me of Chinese Egg Foo Yong.

Quinoa is so versatile, plus it's packed with plant proteins. One-quarter cup has 6 grams of protein. It's a quick fix, too; only 15 minutes cooking time. Here's a website that offers great quinoa recipes[230] like quinoa tabbouleh, quinoa burgers, quinoa and roasted pepper chili, plus 27 other exciting quinoa dishes.

Sorghum

Bob's Red Mill has interesting recipes for making all sorts of goodies with sorghum flour[231] like brownies, pound cake, maple oat nut cookies, scones, and whole grain waffles. Sorghum is the go-to-substitute-for-wheat-flour when baking goodies and treats. You even can make a birthday cake using the pound cake recipe: slice it to make a double or triple layer cake and use a safe frosting between layers. Here's a website

---

228 http://www.drweil.com/drw/u/ART03188/How-to-Cook-Oats.html accessed 3-18-16
229 http://www.southernliving.com/food/entertaining/flavored-butter-recipes/lemon-herb-butter
230 http://www.cookinglight.com/food/recipe-finder/cooking-with-quinoa/buffalo-quinoa-burgers-1 accessed 3-18-16
231 http://www.bobsredmill.com/recipes/ingredient/sorghum-flour/ accessed 3-18-16

for cake frostings[232] that just may fit the bill for that special occasion cake.

Montina Indian Rice Grass

This is a grass not related to rice, which has not been modified, and comes as a mixed baking flour blend ready to use for gluten-free baking[233]. The mixture contains rice flour, tapioca flour, and Montina Pure.

I've listed a wide variety of gluten-free grains and products because many individuals are gluten-intolerant, and those who cook for them can be at a loss as where to find substitutes. Additionally, there's a little tip I'd like to leave with cooks regarding cooking whole grains. If you don't have broth to cook the grains for added flavor, here's a simple yet tasty suggestion: For every cup of water used to cook the grain, add 1 teaspoon of Braggs Amino Acids—gluten-free and organic. The flavor reminds you of vegetable broth, which you didn't have to make ahead of time; peel and chop veggies, and cook for 45 minutes!

Regarding grains, I feel all grain flours should be avoided as much as possible and eat only whole grains or sprouted grains for better nutrition and digestibility of grain sugars and starches.

It is my opinion that some whole grain should be eaten with each meal—not very much—a half a cup will do, because the starches in whole grains are necessary for the microbiota colonies in your intestinal tract to feed off and thrive. Did you know that? They love the fiber and certain starches—"digestive resistant"[234]—in whole grains, which milled and chemicalized flours probably lack. The recommendation

---

232 https://elanaspantry.com/category/toppings/ accessed 3-18-16
233 https://www.azurestandard.com/shop/product/770/ accessed 3-18-16
234 http://advances.nutrition.org/content/4/6/587.full accessed 3-18-16

for digestive resistant starch consumption is six grams per MEAL for health benefits.

Whole grains such as steel cut oats and quinoa are dietary grain recommendations for diabetics.

There are a lot more grains to eat besides wheat. Explore and enjoy them; they're delicious.

Before I leave this chapter, I have a message for those of the Christian faith who participate in receiving communion and are gluten-intolerant: There are gluten-free wafers[235]. Some wafer suppliers certify their products are gluten free, kosher, non-GMO, and free of specific food allergens.

You may want to bring that information to the attention of your congregation.

---

235 http://www.nydailynews.com/life-style/health/gluten-free-communion-wafers-popular-church-article-1.2057402 accessed 3-18-16

Ice Cream That Can Be Nutritious

Certainly, everyone remembers being a kid and loving ice cream cones and popsicles. When I was a youngster, kids used to shout, "I scream, you scream, we all scream for ice cream," while running to the ice cream truck that made the neighborhood rounds on hot summer evenings. Those were the days—in the 1940s—before all the junk ingredients in ice cream, including artificial sweeteners.

Today, frozen dairy and non-dairy desserts are made with all sorts of non-natural and chemical ingredients, which are not healthful, and definitely contribute other toxins to the body's ever-growing toxic burden.

However, there is an ingenious way of making what amounts to imitation ice cream using a fruit, which vegans have been doing for ages, or so it seems. It's frozen banana "ice cream," a one-ingredient recipe that's rather easy but requires a few steps to get the proper consistency.

Personally, when done just right, not only is it delicious and nutritious, but it can pass as banana ice cream, sans the dairy.

Keeping in mind the nutritional values in bananas, especially several B vitamins (2, 3, 6, 9), rich in potassium, plus fiber and even some plant protein, there should be no guilt complex while indulging in frozen banana *pretend* ice cream—with absolutely no added sugars, too.

That easy to eat tropical treat is not a one-trick dessert pony, either. It can be used to make another equally delicious frozen treat that really hits home with both kids and adults—it's a frozen banana on a stick coated with organic chocolate and, if you like, rolled in chopped toasted almonds or raw walnuts. Wow! Chocolate-covered-frozen bananas are easy to make and here's a recipe.

Chocolate-covered Frozen Banana

Make certain the banana has a fair amount of brown spots on the skin, but not overly ripe as it won't hold its form. Peel the banana and insert a wooden skewer almost half-way into one end of the banana. Place the banana on a wax paper-lined cookie sheet and put it into the freezer to freeze solid, about 2 hours. Before taking the banana out of the freezer for its chocolate coating, prepare melted *organic chocolate* according to package instructions and also chop the nuts for sprinkling on the chocolate coating.

Chocolate-Nut Coating

Nuts add even more guilt-free nutrition: B and other vitamins, heart-healthy fats, minerals, and plant protein.

Place the melted chocolate into a dish (corn-on-the-cob type or one that will allow you to roll the banana to coat all sides with chocolate).
Have chopped nuts spread out on a separate piece of wax paper.
Immediately after the banana's chocolate bath, roll it in the nuts on the wax paper, coating all sides.
Transfer to another wax-paper-covered cookie sheet and place into the freezer.

Once frozen solid, you can wrap the frozen banana in wax paper and place it in a freezer bag, flat in the freezer to enjoy later.

The above recipe can be done in a production-line fashion so that you can make and have several treats in the freezer instead of buying junk at the grocery store. Also, I suggest cutting the banana in half before beginning the process, as that will make "kid-size" treats, since many bananas are rather large.

Naked frozen bananas, or those without chocolate and nuts, will work well as treats for those who want plain frozen banana pops.

Frozen Banana Mock Ice Cream
Note: To make this type of "ice cream," cooks need a special kitchen appliance that will process the frozen banana into the consistency needed. It doesn't work very well using a kitchen blender. These kitchen appliances can make sorbets without sugar, just ripe fruit, and manufacturers provide recipes too. There are several brands of frozen dessert makers available, especially online. Prices range from $30 to $99, depending upon one's preference. Some are labeled as "Frozen Fruit Dessert Makers." If you have kiddies and want to get them off ice cream, this kitchen gadget ought to do the trick. Watch the kids having fun making frozen banana ice cream or fruit sorbet!

Recipe for a Frozen Banana Sundae
Process a frozen banana according to a Frozen Fruit Dessert Maker's directions
Place it in a fancy sherbet or ice cream dish and add some chopped toasted almonds, coconut nibs, and organic unsweetened cocoa nibs. Wow!

Toppings for Frozen Banana Ice Cream

Chopped walnuts dry or wet [To make wet walnuts, marinate walnut pieces in organic maple syrup (B grade) in a glass jar with a lid and refrigerate]
Organic unsweetened cocoa/chocolate nibs
Roasted unsalted peanuts, chopped
Chopped pistachio nuts
Toasted almond pieces
Coconut nibs
Chia seeds

Enjoy!

The Mineral Iron

*A*re you aware that there are two sources of dietary iron? One, heme, which is from animal sources and the other source, non-heme, is from plant-based foods.

Animal sources of heme-iron include: beef, chicken, cod, flounder, oysters, pork, salmon, shrimp, tuna, and turkey.

Plant-based non-heme sources of iron include: almonds, apricots, baked beans, black beans, black eye peas, bread made with enriched flour, broccoli, dates, grits, kidney beans, lentils, lima beans, molasses, navy beans, oatmeal, peas, pinto beans, prunes, raisins, rice: brown and white, soybeans, spinach, and tofu.

The amount of iron in milligrams received[236] depends upon the portion size eaten. For animal protein, the average portion size is 3 ounces, while for plant-based foods it depends upon a serving size of one-half to a full cup.

The Daily Value (DV) of iron for a 2,000 calorie diet for adults 19 to 50 years of age is 18 milligrams. However, both male and female adults 50 years and older need only 8 milligrams of iron a day,

---

236 http://www.mckinley.illinois.edu/handouts/dietary_sources_iron.html accessed 1-14-2016

per the NIH. During pregnancy, females need at least 27 milligrams of iron a day. I offer that females during their menstruating years should be certain to maintain a diet rich in iron foods.

The importance of iron should not be underestimated. In addition to providing for the transfer of oxygen from the lungs to tissues, it is necessary for growth, normal cellular functioning, and the synthesis of some hormones and connective tissue.

Iron supplementation, as found in vitamin and mineral pills, sometimes can lead to an overload of iron, which can cause a liver disease called hemochromatosis. Bioavailability of iron is a crucial factor in either a deficiency or an overload. Animal source heme is utilized by the body more efficiently than non-heme plant form. That's why vegetarians and vegans, especially, are told to take vitamin B12 (cobalamin) supplements to make certain iron works efficiently in the body to avoid iron-deficiency anemia. Inflammatory disorders in the body also can interfere with proper iron levels.

Since the main absorption of iron takes place in the duodenum of the small intestine, one has to exercise care about not contracting a duodenal ulcer, which can be caused by the bacterium H. Pylori.

One of the most efficient ways to absorb iron is to eat whole foods organically grown that contain it, as the other nutrients in those foods make iron digestion and absorption easier, plus much more gentle on the stomach than iron supplement pills.

Foods that contain iron include: chickpeas, kidney beans, lentils, liver, most animal meats, oysters, pumpkin seeds, quinoa, soybeans, and spinach (cooked)

M-E-A-T: Do you really want to know what happens to it?

Coincidentally, and almost as if by some providential gift to this writer, the Internet ran a twenty-page series titled "19 Reasons Why You Might Want to Stop Buying Supermarket Meat"[237], which I could not resist including in this book. Why? Because most eaters really aren't aware of what goes on with food raising, processing, and merchandising that, literally, can affect your health.

Furthermore, I'm of the opinion that once an individual is aware of real and serious issues surrounding things that affect us, we are more willing either to listen to reason and facts, and/or make necessary changes to correct them for better outcomes all around.

With that statement in mind, let's consider why you might want to stop buying *supermarket* meat.

Here are the reasons listed by Dan Myers in the above Internet article along with his suggestion that you may want to consider purchasing your meats in an *organic* butcher shop[238]!

---

[237] http://www.msn.com/en-us/health/nutrition/19-reasons-why-you-might-want-to-stop-buying-supermarket-meat/ss-CCiY8Y accessed 1-9-2016

[238] http://www.thedailymeal.com/america-s-25-best-butcher-shops/102413 accessed 1-9-2016

1. The deli slicer is one of the dirtiest places in the supermarket.
2. The packages of raw meat can be E.coli farms.
3. The fish may be mislabeled.
4. Expiration dates on meat packaging are generally meaningless.
5. Meat in the circular is most likely actually not on sale.
6. It's [meat] full of antibiotics.
7. Almost half contain staph bacteria.
8. Some is 'mechanically tenderized', which can be dangerous.
9. Supermarket chickens are pumped with potentially dangerous drugs.
10. A surprising chemical is used to make meat look pink. Myers claims that *"as much as 70 percent of all raw meat sold in supermarkets is treated with a surprising chemical: carbon monoxide."* Why? Because it makes it pink!
11. The vast majority of ground turkey is contaminated with fecal bacteria.
12. If it smells, or is slimy, throw it away.
13. Ground beef can contain meat from hundreds of cows.
14. Ground beef is usually from retired dairy or breeding cows.
15. You should look for the USDA shield on the packaging.
16. Contaminated chicken and turkey sickens 200,000 Americans yearly with salmonella.
17. A new law[239] makes it legal for supermarket meat to not be labeled with the country of origin.
18. Thanksgiving [frozen] turkeys could have been slaughtered years ago. Myers suggests getting a pasture-raised turkey from a local or organic farmer or butcher.
19. Supermarket-bound turkeys may suffer more than any other animal. They are forced to grow so unnaturally fast that they suffer from broken bones, breathing problems, and congestive heart failure from stacking on 20 to 40 pounds in 12 to 19 weeks! Basically, you are eating a sick bird.

---

239 http://www.thedailymeal.com/cook/congress-repeals-country-origin-labeling-meat-effective-immediately/010516 accessed 1-9-2016

Now, let's juxtapose the above information with pasture-raised food animals.

Pasture-raised animals eat the grass that grows under their feet! Usually, they are raised on local farms and are treated humanely at every stage of life. They are not – or should not be – fed growth hormones or synthetic feeds or injected with synthetic hormones to produce milk. The only time they can be treated with antibiotics is if they get sick.

Statistically, a factory-farmed cow must consume 8 pounds of grain to yield one pound of meat! It is estimated that up to almost one-third of feed lot cattle develop liver abscesses from their high-grain diet. What does that do to the quality of the meat those animals produce? I hope those animals' livers are not sold for human consumption.

Cows (beef), as designed by Nature, are grass-eaters. Consequently, soy and corn—especially GMO crops with all the glyphosate residues in them—raise the acidity levels in their bodies making them more prone to illnesses, E.coli, and other bacterial infections, I contend.

However, as Mike Adams claims, *"The economics of raising meat with cheap inputs has made heavy grain diets standard with most livestock, even when other diets are more natural choices. The drive to find the cheapest inputs for feed rations makes subsidized, genetically modified corn and soybean feed the most popular choice, with smaller amounts of hay, forage, or by-product added in. Typically drenched in pesticides and cheaply produced for fodder, ethanol, or junk food production, these crops often have contaminants that, when consumed by livestock, enter into our food supply."* [240]

---

240 Mike Adams, *Food Forensics,* (Dallas, TX: BenBellaBooks, 2016), Pp. 149-150.

Pasture-raised beef is lower in total fat, higher in vitamins along with a healthier ratio of Omega-3 and Omega-6 fatty acids than conventional, industrial farming meat and dairy products.

CAFO (Concentrated Animal Feeding Operation) is the term given to huge factory farms that raise cattle almost as if an assembly line production rather than dealing with living, sensitive animals.

Chickens scratch in dirt to find and eat bugs and grass, not cooped up in "high rise" hen houses never to see the light of day. Chickens and pigs need some grain in their diets, but they are not fed GMO grain.

Free-range, grass-fed chickens have 30 percent less saturated fat and 28 percent fewer calories than factory-farmed poultry. Pasture-raised hens lay eggs with 10 percent less fat, 40 percent more vitamin A, and 400 percent more Omega-3 fatty acids!

Pastured pork (hogs) produce meat 18 to 291 percent higher in Omega-3 fatty acids, since they are not given corn and soybean meal, which are high in Omega-6 polyunsaturated fats. The more Omega-6s in hog chow, the more they produce in their meat, proving at animal level, "You are what you eat."

One farmer, Joel Salatin of Polyface Farms[241] in rural Swope, Virginia, has become the "face and voice" of sustainable agriculture and pasture-raised cattle and poultry. His family has been raising food animals sustainably on the same farm without chemicals added for close to a hundred years. I had the extreme good fortune to spend one glorious September Saturday a few years ago visiting Polyface Farm, riding the hay wagon for a grand tour of the opera-

---

241 https://www.youtube.com/watch?feature=player_detailpage&v=KxTfQpv8xGA#t=179 accessed 2-17-16

tion, and then enjoying an organically-grown exquisite luncheon. With every food item coming from the farm, I had no problem with all the wonderful vegetable dishes, but I must admit I ate some raw milk cheese and went back for a couple of servings of homemade raw milk, honey vanilla ice cream. Food tastes that I can't explain, and so unbelievably fresh and nutritious.

After the meat leaves the slaughter house, it's subjected to numerous chemical insults that, in my opinion, are not necessary and ought to make it unfit for human consumption. One such example is the addition of nitrates or nitrites, which essentially turn into nitrosamines and nitrosamides[242] that may contribute to colon tumors and gastrointestinal cancers, but there seems to be no definitive correlation to confirm that. Sodium nitrate is thought to damage blood vessels thereby leading to heart disease.

Many meat sausages, hot dogs, and luncheon meats are made with nitrates or nitrites. Nitrates and nitrites are approved by and subject to FDA and USDA regulations for bacon, bologna, corned beef, hot dogs, luncheon meats, sausages, canned and cured meat, and hams. However, it's what happens to them during the digestive processes – the conversion to nitrosamines and nitrosamides – that present a problem.

According to the data I was able to find, the following contain higher amounts of nitrates than other foods: bacon, chicken liver pâté, corned beef, ham, hot dogs, liver pâté, luncheon meats, red sausages (*Saveloys*), and smoked meat.

Nitrosamines are in bacon, fish: pickled—salted—smoked, pork, and salami.

---

242 http://www.ncbi.nlm.nih.gov/pubmed/922686 accessed 3-9-16

However, there are brands that offer nitrate- and nitrite-free meats. Applegate[243] Natural and Organic Meats is a brand offering GMO-free and nitrate-free meats and available in supermarkets.

According to Mike Adams,

In December in 2015, the FDA withdrew its approval of Nitarsone for use in chicken feed, stating, "Following this action, there are no FDA-approved, arsenic-based drugs for use in food producing animals."
http://www.fda.gov/AnimalVeterinary/NewsEvents/CVMUpdates/ucm440668.htm [244]

Regarding industrialized fish farming, Adams talks about how fish are gendered:

Worse, the use of hormones to manipulate sex ratios and promote maturation has become dominant in aquatic farming for food production. Researchers say that nearly all fish bred in captivity have reproductive dysfunction, prompting those raising fish to administer reproductive hormones, with various possible effects not only on the fish, but on those who consume it.936 Control of water temperature and the administration of hormone therapy are often necessary to achieve commercially desirable reproduction. Luteinizing hormones (LH) and gonadotropin-release hormones (GnRHa) are often administered, while interrupting normal spawning behavior under captive aquaculture conditions may also require artificial forms of fertilization.937 Sex-inversed males, altered via hormone treatments, are frequently used in fish farming to fertilize female stocks for consumption for many species including trout and tilapia.938 Studies show that some of these hormones, which can disrupt the

---
243 http://www.applegate.com/ accessed 3-9-16
244 Mike Adams, *Food Forensics*, (Dallas, TX: BenBellaBooks, 2016), Pg. 157.

endocrine system, end up in wastewater, groundwater, and even drinking water supplies.[245]

If you're going to eat fish, "wild caught" may be another choice, depending upon where it's been caught, since Fukushima radiation is impacting sea life in the Pacific Ocean. [246]

Resources

Organic meats, milk could have more of good-for-you fats, study finds
http://edition.cnn.com/2016/02/18/health/organic-meat-milk-fatty-acids-omega-3s/index.html

Newcastle University study: "New study finds clear differences between organic and non-organic milk and meat" February 15, 2016
https://www.sciencedaily.com/releases/2016/02/160215210707.htm

---

245 Mike Adams, *Food Forensics,* (Dallas, TX: BenBellaBooks, 2016), Pg. 158.
246 http://www.naturalnews.com/049446_Pacific_Ocean_fisheries_Fukushima_radiation.html accessed 3-16-16

Medicinal Mushrooms: Fact or fiction?

Mushrooms have been considered and used as a medicinal treatment as far back as anyone seems to remember, particularly by practitioners of Traditional Chinese Medicine (TCM), Tibetan, and Ayurveda practitioners going back millennia[247]. Even the five-thousand-year-old mummified Ice Man Otzi, whose intact skeleton was found in 1991 on the alpine Similaun glacier between Italy and Austria (altitude 3210 meters), had several mushrooms in his pouch. Scientists identified them as two different types of polypores: One was a tinder fungus and the other was a medicinal birch, which has been used in eliminating worms. Interestingly, Otzi's 'autopsy' indicated that he had a whipworm intestinal parasite.

Even Hippocrates mentioned the healing powers of mushrooms for certain ailments. However, Pliny and Galen did not hold mushrooms in high esteem. That sentiment may still be alive in some segments of the healing arts, since they are fungi and some look upon them with disdain.

Below is a listing of mushrooms[248] -- some valued for their medicinal properties, others for their wonderfully delicious tastes.

---
247 http://www.ncbi.nlm.nih.gov/pmc/articles/PMC3121254/ accessed 1-7-2016
248 http://www.medicalmushrooms.net/ accessed 1-7-2016

Birch Bracket / Kanbatake / Piptoporus Betulinus   [not recommended for cooking; use as a medicinal]
This mushroom, aka birch polypore, is an anti-inflammatory. It's a very effective anti-viral, plus being an intestinal parasite cleanser. It can be used as an anti-tumor and immune enhancer. They make great medicinal teas. Here's an interesting video taken in a birch forest that shows and explains these wonderful mushrooms.
https://www.youtube.com/watch?v=3pOyHZHfKfo&feature=player_embedded#t=567.

Cauliflower mushroom / Hanabiratake / Sparassis Crispa
This leafy-like mushroom contains sparassol, an anti-fungal and natural antibiotic. It also contains beta-glucans, which slow tumor growth, and stimulate the immune system. It's not readily available in the marketplace. Since it grows wild, and is not commercially cultivated, it has a unique earthy taste. A cauliflower mushroom can grow as large as several pounds!

Nutrient Content: B vitamins and various minerals, like most mushrooms. However, I could not find a specific listing for the cauliflower mushroom nutrients.

Chaga / Kabanoanatake / Inonotus obliquus
This super mushroom grows on birch trees and usually is consumed as a tea. It has a super-abundance of beta-D-glucans, which help the immune system. It works well with chemotherapy treatments. It helps normalize blood pressure and cholesterol levels. Its polysaccharides promote healthy blood sugar levels. It also contains Superoxide Dismutase (SOD), which protects against free radicals, and is an anti-inflammatory.

Nutrient Content: B vitamins including B2 and B3, flavonoids, phenol, Superoxide Dismutase (SOD), an enzyme that halts oxidation and free radical formation. Minerals: copper, calcium, potassium, manganese, zinc, and iron.

Chestnut mushroom / Brown Caps / Yanagimatsutake / Agrocybe Aegerita

The chestnut mushroom can be mistaken for Cremini or "Baby Portobello" mushrooms because of their color and size. These mushrooms are rich in antioxidants and help suppress high cholesterol levels. They are thought to help prevent breast and prostate cancers and bone loss caused by osteoporosis. However, they are not readily available commercially.

Nutrient content: Vitamins B1, B2, B3, B6, B9, pantothenic acid, C, E

Minerals: iron, phosphorus, magnesium, copper, selenium, potassium, sodium, sulfur, zinc

Common mushroom / Button or White mushroom / Agaricus Bisporus

This is the most commonly eaten mushroom, especially by westerners. Research on common mushrooms indicates that they, too, have medicinal properties. Mushrooms can improve eyesight, hearing, circulation, impotency, migraine headaches, and reduce infections. Mushrooms contain CLA (conjugated linoleic acid), which reduces the detrimental effects of high levels of estrogen. They provide protection against inflammation. They contain a powerful antioxidant, L-Ergothioneine, which scavenges free radicals and helps protect against DNA damage.

Nutrient Content: Plant protein Vitamins: B1, B2, B3, B5, B6, B9, B12, C, provitamin D (Ergosterol), choline, betaine Minerals: calcium, iron, magnesium, phosphorus, potassium, sodium, zinc, copper, selenium

Cordyceps sinensis / Caterpillar fungus / Tochukasu [a medicinal mushroom, not for cooking]

This mushroom has tremendously powerful anti-cancer properties. It's been known to reduce cholesterol levels. In TCM these mushrooms are considered to benefit lungs and kidneys. It's comparable to a "super ginseng" to rejuvenate the body. Studies have proven it benefits the cardiovascular system. It's effective for adrenals, asthma, bronchitis, libido, and tinnitus. It's an anti-inflammatory, anti-viral, and anti-bacterial.

Nutrient Content: Vitamins: B1, B12, C Minerals: Trace elements Amino acids/protein, nucleic acids, and polysaccharides beta 1,3 glucan

Enokitake / Enoki / Snow puff mushroom / Flammulina Populicola

Commonly referred to as Enoki mushrooms, they look like tiny lollipops. However, they are packed with nutrients such as B vitamins, some plant proteins, and a substantial amount of beta-glucan.

Health benefits include immune boosting, weight loss, maintain proper blood sugar levels, lower blood lipids, and enhanced metabolic processes in the body.

Nutrient Content: Vitamins: B1, B2, B3, B5, B9, provitamin D (Ergosterol) Minerals: calcium, potassium, phosphorus, iron, copper, selenium Antioxidants

God's mushroom / Mushroom of the sun / Himematsutake / Agaricus blazei [medicinal mushroom, not for cooking]

Traditionally, this mushroom was used to treat atherosclerosis, hepatitis, diabetes, dermatitis, and cancer. It contains a unique beta-glucan complex, which seems to activate the immune system, including T-lymphocytes. As a supplement, its use is "antitumor." It's also known as an anti-viral. Increase in NK (natural killer) blood cells.

Nutrient Content: Vitamins B1, B2, B3   Minerals: calcium and iron
The highest beta-glucan content of any mushroom: Beta-1,3-D-glucan, Beta 1,4-a-D-glucan, and Beta 1,6-D-glucan

King Oyster / French horn / Pleurotus Eryngii

This mushroom contains a natural statin compound, Lovastatin. It also has nutritional/medicinal properties that improve blood levels, hemoglobin in particular. It's known as an anti-inflammatory and good source of antioxidants.

Nutrient Content: B vitamins, provitamin D (Ergosterol), proteins, iron

Lion's Mane / Hedgehog mushroom / Yamabushitake / Hericium erinaceus

This mushroom has been used in the treatment of digestive tract ailments. It, too, has immune boosting properties and can stimulate production of Nerve Growth Factor, which is necessary for neurological sensory neurons growth. There's the possibility that it can protect the myelin sheath of nerves. It contains 15 percent beta-glucans.

Nutrient Content: 16 Amino acids, including 7 essential amino acids Vitamins: carotene, B1, B2   Minerals: phosphorus, iron, calcium

Maitake / Hen of the woods / Huishuhua

This mushroom is best known for its ability to reduce the side effects of cancer chemotherapy.

Maitake beta-glucan has been shown to inhibit tumor grow effectively 80 percent of the time. Maitake mushrooms support the immune function. It contains beta-1,3 glucan and beta-1,6 glucan. It also helps in high blood pressure treatment, liver disease, and as an antioxidant.

As a supplement, its use is for breast and prostate cancer, and HIV. Maitake mushrooms have been eaten for over three thousand years by the Chinese and Japanese.

Nutrient Content: Amino acids: Alanine, Arginine, Asparagine, Glutamine, Lysine, Serine, Threonine, Valine Vitamins: B1, B2, C, provitamin D (Ergosterol), E Minerals: selenium, potassium, phosphorus, magnesium, calcium, sodium, zinc

Oyster / Hiratake / Pleurotus Ostreatus

Oyster mushrooms are an all-around food for maintaining all body systems in good health. They help in the metabolism of fats and reduce the production of low density lipoproteins (LDLs) the "bad" cholesterol. They can help lower blood pressure and stimulate blood circulation.

Nutrient Content: 18 Amino Acids, especially Taurine and Glutamic acid. Vitamins: B1, B2, B3, C, provitamin D (Ergosterol) Minerals: phosphorus, potassium, zinc, copper, molybdenum, calcium, iron, magnesium, manganese, selenium, sodium

Reishi / Lingshi / Ganoderma Lucidum

The Reishi mushroom has over two thousand years of documented medicinal history in China and Japan, used as a tea. The Red Reishi mushroom improves liver function. Due to its various types of polysaccharides, Reishi mushroom enhances the immune system, especially several interleukins. It's been used in the treatment of hypertension and hypercholesterolemia. Chinese studies indicate substantial improvement for chronic bronchitis patients. It has anti-inflammatory effects and has been used to treat diabetes, hepatitis C, and respiratory problems. As a supplement, its use is for anti-inflammatory, antiviral, hepatitis, HIV, immune system, and cancer.

Nutrient Content: Amino acids, fatty acids Minerals: potassium, iron, magnesium, manganese, zinc, calcium, copper, sodium

Shiitake / Forest Mushroom / Lentinula Edodes

Shiitake mushrooms have a medicinal history of more than one thousand years! It's been used to treat cardiovascular disease, colds, and flu. It has properties that greatly enhance the immune system and has been used as an adjunct cancer therapy.

The Shiitake mushroom contains 18% plant-based proteins, plus potassium, niacin, calcium, magnesium, phosphorus, and B vitamins. It contains anti-viral properties and has compounds that inhibit tumors in research animals. It contains 10 percent beta glucan polysaccharides: 1,3 beta-D-glucan and beta-1,6-D-glucopyranoside. As a supplement, its use is antimicrobial, cholesterol, and immune support.

Nutrient Content: Amino acids: Isoleucine, Leucine, Lysine, Methionine, Phenylalanine, Threonine, Tryptophan, and Valine—all essential amino acids Vitamins: B1, B2, B3, B12, C, D Minerals: iron, zinc, manganese, potassium, phosphorus

There are several other mushrooms, which are used as healing supplements or remedies, but aren't appropriate for use in cooking.

Deadly Poisonous Mushrooms

One thing I must caution you about is that mushrooms can be deceptive in their looks and be extremely poisonous, especially those growing in the wild. If you don't know how to *correctly* identify mushrooms, please do not forage for them nor eat them. You can wind up very sick or even dead. Some wild mushrooms are extremely toxic. The beautiful *Amanita Muscaria*, commonly called "Fly Agaric" or "Fly Amanita," probably is the most toxic of all mushrooms, yet it is exquisitely beautiful. All Amanita mushrooms are deadly poisonous: *The Death Cap, Amanita Caesarea, Amanita Pantherina, Amanita Virosa, Penny Bun, Amanita Hemibapha*—just to name a few.

Stick with commercially, organically-grown mushrooms, and reliable sources of mushroom supplements, if you choose to go that route.

Most mushrooms start out as mycelium—thread- and root-like *hyphae* that actually are the vegetative part of the fungus, which usually grow subterraneously and send up a "fruit body," the familiar mushroom that is harvested either to eat or processed into a medicinal extract. Supplemental forms of mushrooms can be in the form of mycelium biomass, mycelium powder, and two types of mushroom extracts—hydro-alcohol and hot water.

Mushrooms long-chain of simple sugars polysaccharides is the key to their immune-modulating effects in the human body.

Mushrooms, especially the 'meaty' ones like French horn, Maitake, and Shiitake, also can become a great dietary support food during the transition time of eating less meat. Those three mushrooms have a tactile sensation in the mouth that resembles some meats or seafood, e.g., lobster.

Resource
Are Medicinal Mushrooms Safe?
http://mykosan.com/medicinal-mushroom-safety-information/

Medicinal Mushroom Recipes

Shiitake-Maitake Stir Fry
2 Tbsp. EV olive oil
½ sweet onion, chopped
½ large sweet red pepper, chopped
8 broccoli florets broken into smaller florets

1 carrot, sliced
8 Shiitake mushrooms, stems removed and sliced into strips
½ cup Maitake mushrooms, chopped coarsely
OR substitute Baby Bella mushrooms if you can't find fresh Maitake mushrooms
2 cloves garlic, minced
1 inch thin piece of fresh ginger, peeled and minced
¼ lb. firm tofu, cut into small cubes (optional)
2 Tbsp. Braggs Amino Acids
½ tsp. toasted sesame oil
1 bunch scallions, thinly sliced

Heat the oil in a 10 inch stainless steel fry pan or wok
Add onions and sauté on medium heat for 1 minute
Add red pepper, broccoli, carrot, mushrooms, garlic, and ginger and sauté on medium heat 4 to 5 minutes, stirring constantly
Add Braggs Amino Acids, sesame oil, and tofu cubes
Stir well and cook until tofu is heated through; only 1 or 2 minutes on medium heat
Garnish with scallions
Additional garnish could be 1 Tbsp. of toasted black or brown sesame seeds

Serving suggestion
Serve over steamed brown, wild, or mixed blend of rice or cooked quinoa.

Mushroom Miso Soup (Gluten-free)
1 quart/liter water
5 large Shiitake mushrooms, stems removed and cut into strips
2 small French trumpet/horn mushrooms, sliced OR 6 small Baby Bella mushrooms, sliced

1 inch fresh ginger, peeled and scored
1 garlic clove, cut in half
Pinch of cayenne pepper
1 cup fresh baby spinach leaves [OR ½ cup kale, chopped small]
2 Tbsp. Braggs Amino Acids
¼ tub (4 oz.) firm tofu, small dice
1 heaping tsp garbanzo bean miso with 3 Tbsp. soup broth mixed into a paste
1 bunch scallions, thin slice

Into a soup pot place water, mushrooms, ginger, garlic, cayenne pepper and bring to a boil.
Turn to medium heat and cook for 10 minutes.
Add spinach leaves [kale], Braggs Amino Acids and cook on medium heat for 3 minutes.
Add tofu and miso paste; mix very well and cook on low heat for 3 minutes.
Turn off heat and add scallions. Mix well and serve.

Suggested serving:
Serve with a side portion of steamed brown, wild, or red rice, or combination of all. Garnish with toasted sesame seeds or *Gomasio* (a macrobiotic condiment found in health food stores, co-ops, and some supermarkets).
You can reheat soup, but do not boil it.

Smoothies: A fresh start to your day

Everyone is familiar with luscious smoothie drinks as a nice picker-upper or snack drink, but did you ever think of drinking a nutrition-packed smoothie for breakfast? That's how I often start a day—with an organic apple juice—especially fresh apple cider in season—blended with other organic fruits. The smoothies I will share with you are jammed packed with enzymes, vitamins, and minerals without man-made chemicals when you choose organically grown fruits and berries[249].

The smoothies I like to make use organic apples, organic bananas, organic blackberries, organic raspberries, and organic strawberries. Nutritionally, those fruit-and-berries smoothies stack up as powerhouses of nutrition. *However, these Smoothies should not be eaten by diabetics!* Diabetics must get their blood sugar normalized, which can be done with proper medical supervision using holistic medical practices[250] and diet[251], before they can enjoy the nutritional benefits of several fruits in a smoothie, I definitely suggest.

---

[249] http://www.naturalhealth365.com/berries-prevent-cancer-1777.html accessed 3-17-16
[250] http://treeoflifecenterus.com/retreat/diabetes-recovery-program/ accessed 1-23-16
[251] http://www.amazon.com/There-Cure-Diabetes-Revised-Edition/dp/158394544X accessed 1-23-16

Apples, depending upon variety, can contain between 1 and 10 percent of the Daily Values of most vitamins except vitamin D. They contain numerous minerals: calcium, magnesium, iron, phosphorus, potassium, and sodium; a fair amount of phytosterols (lower cholesterol, especially LDL, and act as immunostimulants), Omega-3 and -6 fatty acids, a negligible amount of protein, and fruit sugars. Their estimated glycemic load is 3.

Bananas when ripe, i.e., brown spots on its skin, are digestible and contain very generous Daily Values of all the B-complex vitamins except B-12, plus lesser amount of vitamins A, C, E, and K. Bananas are extraordinarily generous with potassium, manganese, and magnesium, and supply calcium, iron, phosphorus, sodium, zinc, copper, and selenium. They contain phytosterols, Omega-3 and -6 fatty acids, a nice amount of protein, plus sugars and starches. Their estimated glycemic load is low – 18!

Blackberries are a rich source of vitamins C and K; supply a fair amount of folate (B9); the B-complex vitamins, except B12; and vitamins A and E. The minerals they supply include generous amounts of manganese and copper with respectable amounts of calcium, iron, magnesium, phosphorus, potassium, zinc, and selenium along with Omega-3 and -6 fatty acids, and some protein. They provide a generous supply of fiber. Their estimated glycemic load is 4.

Raspberries are such a delicious treat to eat, plus jam-packed with nutrition. They contain a generous supply of the Daily Value for vitamin C and vitamin K, with lesser amounts of vitamins A, E, and the B-complex, except no B12. Mineral-wise, raspberries are a generous source of manganese and provide other minerals like calcium, iron, magnesium, phosphorus, potassium, zinc, and copper, with negligible sodium. They supply generous amounts of Omega-3 and -6 fatty acids, some protein, and sugars. Their estimated glycemic load is 3. And they taste so good too!

However, there's something to be concerned about with red raspberries: they have a proclivity to develop black spots, which are mold or fungal growths, *which should not be eaten.* Fresh raspberries should be eaten very shortly after purchasing and not allowed to sit in the refrigerator for days, in my opinion. I buy enough for only two days and devour them while at their peak quality and flavor.

Strawberries really are the berries! Everyone loves them and with good reason. They are filled with nutrition: high in vitamin C; generous in folic acid (B9, folate); and contain the B-complex vitamins except B12; vitamins A, E, and K. They have very respectable amounts of Omega-3 and -6 fatty acids, phytosterols, sugars, and their estimated glycemic load is 3.

Berries and apples, too, are rich in antioxidants, which fight disease and prevent cellular damage. Anthocyanins are the antioxidants that give *strawberries* their red color.

Raspberries are really blessed with generous amounts of phenolic flavonoids such as anthocyanins, ellagic acid or tannin, quercetin, gallic acid, cyanidins, pelargonidins, catechins, kaempferol, and salicylic acid. Those antioxidants are thought to play nutritional roles against ageing, cancer, inflammation, and neuro-degenerative diseases. So, you can see why I came up with a few smoothie recipes that not only are filling, but act like a delicious vitamin and mineral pill. To make certain I get enough balanced nutrition while drinking my breakfast, I eat a couple handfuls of refrigerated, raw jumbo pecans—unsalted and not fried or baked in oil. That breakfast lasts me 4 or more hours, depending upon how much brain power I'm using during research work or writing articles.

Breakfast—or anytime—Smoothie Recipes
A special note about bananas in making Smoothies

The recipes below make about 12 to 14 ounces of Smoothie.

I recommend a small size banana, as opposed to a large banana, and it should have some brown spots on it, too, meaning that starches have started to convert to sugars and are more easily digested.

I usually use 2 or 3 *baby* organic bananas to make my Smoothies. If 'babies' aren't available, then I use the smallest size organic banana I can find at the organic green grocer.

Apple-Banana-Blackberry Smoothie
1 cup organic apple cider or juice
1 organic ripe banana, cut into pieces
20 fresh organic blackberries OR ½ cup frozen blackberries defrosted

Place all ingredients into a blender cup and process a little longer than a minute—the seeds need to be crushed better—until creamy smooth.
Smoothie heaven in a glass!

Apple-Banana-Raspberry Smoothie
1 cup organic apple cider or juice
1 organic ripe banana, cut into pieces
20 fresh organic red raspberries OR ½ cup frozen raspberries defrosted

Place all ingredients into a blender cup and process about 1 full minute until creamy smooth.
Indulge your taste buds in pure delight.

Apple-Banana-Strawberry Smoothie
1 cup organic apple cider or juice
1 organic ripe banana, cut into pieces

4 large or 6 smaller organic strawberries cut in half or ½ cup frozen strawberries defrosted

Place all ingredients into a blender cup and process about 1 full minute until creamy smooth.
What a special treat!

Apple-Banana Smoothie (for when you can't get berries)
1 cup organic apple cider or juice
1 organic ripe banana, cut into pieces
Optional: scant 1/8 tsp organic *Korintje* cinnamon added for a wonderful taste treat

Place ingredients into a blender cup and process about 1 full minute until creamy smooth.
Enjoy this treat anytime.

You probably noticed that I didn't include a Blueberry Smoothie recipe. Well, blueberries just don't make the cut on the taste test, in my opinion, like the other berries do, so I left them out. However, if you want to make a Blueberry Smoothie, just follow the recipe for the Blackberry Smoothie.

Now here's a smoothie-like story from my past—years ago when I was a very young girl during the late 1940s. At that time there were "Banana Milk Shakes" made at home that my family, especially my father loved, which I would be asked to make Saturday nights during TV time, since that was my "specialty" in the kitchen. If I remember correctly, the recipe was promoted on TV—yes we had TV programs back then. The recipe I used called for 1 ripe banana mashed very finely using a dinner fork—blenders weren't common kitchen appliances then—combined with 1 glass of milk and a little bit of vanilla extract.

That milk shake was truly decadent, especially since it was made with non-homogenized milk—the kind with the cream on the top and you would have to shake the milk bottle to disburse the cream throughout the milk. Oh! Was that milk good!

Let's fast forward to 2016, when smoothies are all the rage. I decided to include a different twist on the Banana Milk Shake and call it a *Banana Milk Smoothie*.

Banana Milk Smoothie
1 ripe medium-size banana
1 cup almond or coconut milk (nut milks are compatible with fruit)
Non-dairy milks (oat, rice, soy) are not compatible food combinations with fruit, and can cause digestive distress.
1/8 tsp vanilla extract
Sprinkle of Korintje cinnamon

Combine all ingredients into a blender cup and process until very smooth.

For those who have nut or gluten intolerances, maybe modifying the above recipe to substitute 1 cup of water for almond or coconut milks could work for you.

Soup, the Ultimate Comfort Food

In the mid-1980s, while traveling throughout what was the former Yugoslavia before it was broken up into several countries due to a civil war, I experienced an epiphany about soup, which was other cultures have several definitions and presentations for what I knew as soup.

I vividly remember ordering soup in the hotel dining room where we were staying in Opatija, Yugoslavia—now Croatia, 13 kilometers west of Rijeka, the port city on the Adriatic Sea from which we took the overnight steamer down to Dubrovnik. The waitress kept asking me which type of soup I wanted to order. All I could say was, "Soup, soup!" She asked if I were an American, to which I shook my head yes, and then she proceeded to explain that in their country there were two types of what I generically called soup.

One version was "chorba," a soup chockful of chunky vegetables, almost like a stew but with more liquid, that was served in a large bowl. The other was "zoupa," more like what I'd call consommé and served in a small bowl. Maybe there could be a few sprigs of parsley or some other herbs floating in it. I told her I wanted chorba, and what she served me truly was a gastronomic delight. That was my memorable indoctrination into the variables of what I call soup.

I've enjoyed soup in numerous countries and some of the best soups I can remember eating were in Spain and the Canary Islands: Soups laced with olive oil and savory garlic, cooked to perfection and always served in beautiful dinnerware.

So, what is it about soup that thrills me? Well, I happen to think that soups—especially hearty, warm soups—are the ultimate in comfort food, at least for me. In winter, when it's cold and snowy, soup really knows how to warm you up. In summer, a spicy Gazpacho can cool me down like no ice cream cone could. Anytime in between, I eat soup as often as I can—sometimes twice a day!

Why do I like soup as much as I do? Probably because it's so dog-gone good for you; it's chock full of all kinds of nutrition: vitamins, minerals, enzymes, fiber, broth, plus soup's easy on the digestive system. Also, I can make a potful that will last several days, or I can freeze some in portion-controlled containers.

One of the fundamentals of human nutrition I learned numerous years ago during my studies was about minerals and their importance in human health. Actually, the role of vitamins is to make minerals work in the body! Furthermore, there are metalloenzymes, which are key factors in mineral absorption, especially for zinc. I think just about everyone is familiar with the importance of the mineral calcium in bones. However, the most important mineral for all soft body tissues is potassium, and soups are extremely generous and delicious sources for supplying potassium. Vegetables release their nutrients into the broth, if not cooked at too high a heat that can damage them, and you just slurp up all that tasty nutrition. That's why I often eat soup twice a day; it's so good for my body and health—plus it tastes so good.

Dr Joel Fuhrman, MD, an internationally recognized expert on nutrition, says this about soup:

"Only small amounts of nutrients are lost with conservative cooking like making a soup, but many more nutrients are made more absorbable. These nutrients would have been lost if those vegetables had been consumed raw. When we heat, soften and moisturize the vegetables and beans, we dramatically increase the potential digestibility and absorption of many beneficial and nutritious compounds. We also increase the plant proteins in the diet, especially important for those eating a plant-based diet with limited or no animal products."

For anyone who is determined to regain his/her health, I feel it is most important to eat as many vegetables a day as possible and in as many or varied ways: raw, juiced, baked, steamed, stir-fry, stews, salads, and, of course, soups. I further believe that to maintain a proper acid/alkaline balance, we need to eat more alkaline base foods, which most vegetables are. Also, I eat a minimum of ten vegetables a day – often that many during my dinner meal – and soups are an exceptionally easy way to get as many veggies into your diet without having to use too many pots and pans.

I'd like to encourage you to try eating soup for breakfast instead of pouring yourself a bowl of processed starchy grain cereals with homogenized BST/rBGH cow's milk. The nutritional difference between a soup breakfast and a starchy cereal breakfast is unbelievable—a ten-to-one in favor of soup!

If I have to be on the road early, my standard "travel" day breakfast is a large bowl of homemade vegetable soup spiked with some seaweed served with a side order of steamed mixed brown, wild, and basmati rice, or quinoa topped with a tablespoonful of toasted sesame seeds. That breakfast lasts me up to five hours without feeling hungry and no sugar spikes or let downs.

One of my favorite ways to eat soup is to enjoy a cup of "cream-style" soup before dinner or as an afternoon drink instead of tea, juice, or water. The cream-style soup recipes in this book use no dairy or synthetic creamers, just vegetables cooked and processed in a certain way that makes them cream style, plus absolutely delicious!

Eating for recouping and maintaining health requires establishing a different mindset about food, especially about eating many more vegetables than the average person is used to having on a daily basis, especially in western cultures where steak and fries dominate food choices. Other foods like fruits, nuts, and protein are important, but the most important is plant-based vegetables and the more the variety, the better: leafy greens, cabbage family, tubers and roots, pod vegetables, and sprouts, e.g., alfalfa, broccoli, radish, and watercress.

A special note about my soup recipes

Many recipes below include miso, a fermented food, which is an excellent source for feeding the microbiome of the gut and keeping the intestinal tract supplied with healthy flora colonies to discourage overgrowths of Candida Albicans, the unfortunate downfall of many cancer patients.

I use Miso Master® garbanzo bean miso because that brand is certified gluten-free by the National Sanitation Foundation. Furthermore, I feel better that no GMOs or glyphosate residues are in the miso, as it's made without soy, wheat, or grains—they use chick peas (garbanzo beans), which contain no gluten. Additionally, miso enriches the taste and provides depth to soups, I feel.

Here are some of my favorite soup recipes, which I hope you will try and enjoy as much as I do.

Soup Recipes

Italian Style White Bean Soup
1 ½ quarts or liters of water
1 15 oz. can white beans (Cannellini) not drained
4 celery ribs, chopped
1 large onion, chopped
2 carrots cut in coins
1 small potato, chopped
2 cloves of garlic, finely chopped
1 tsp fresh thyme, chopped (add a little more if you like thyme)
¼ tsp Himalayan pink salt
Pinch or two of cayenne pepper
Slight sprinkling of Chili Powder
¼ cup fresh parsley, chopped
1 Tbsp. extra virgin olive oil

Into a large soup pot with a lid, combine all ingredients except parsley and olive oil
Bring to a boil, and turn heat/fire down to medium low
Cook for 30 minutes with lid on the pot
Remove from heat/fire and add parsley and olive oil
Mix well

Note: When reheating this soup, do not bring to it a boil, as the parsley and olive oil should not be overheated to change the taste or nutrient content.

As a soup topping, *and if you eat cheese,* add a sprinkling of *Parmesan Reggiano* cheese flakes to each bowl of soup for a delightful Italian taste treat.

Chinese Style Vegetable Soup (Gluten-free)
This soup takes very little cooking time, so have all the ingredients prepped and ready to add to the pot. Also, it tastes much better the second day reheated—just don't boil it.

1 ½ quarts or liters water
½ cup green cabbage, chopped
1 cup sweet onion, chopped
10 Shiitake mushrooms, stems removed and chopped
2 medium carrots, chopped
1 inch of fresh ginger, peeled, left whole and scored
2 cloves of garlic cut in half
2 pinches cayenne pepper
2 Tbsp. Braggs Amino Acids [non-GMO soy vegetable protein seasoning]

Combine all the above ingredients into a large soup pot; bring to a boil; turn heat/fire down to medium and cook 10 minutes

Add:
1 cup baby spinach leaves
3 ribs Bok Choy—not baby Bok Choy—chopped and use the leaves
Handful of snow peas, remove ends and strings
Cook on medium low heat 3 to 5 minutes.

Add:
1 tsp Braggs Amino Acids
½ lb. firm tofu, small dice
1 tsp toasted sesame oil
1 bunch scallions, sliced thinly
Immediately turn off heat and mix well.

To Serve:
If you can find organic Chinese dumplings (pot stickers-*there's gluten in them*), place 3 into a flat bottom soup bowl and place 2 or 3 ladlesful of soup on top of dumplings. Pure Chinese style soup!

Gluten-free serving
If *you are gluten-sensitive/intolerant*, serve with a side of steamed brown or mixed brown and wild rice
OR
Gluten-free (rice and millet) cooked *Lotus Foods Rice Ramen Noodles* placed into the soup bowl

Butternut Squash Soup (Gluten-free)
2 heaping cups butternut squash, peeled and chopped
OR 1 20 oz. packaged, precut fresh butternut squash
1 quart or liter + 1 cup water
½ cup onion, diced
1 rib celery, diced
Slight sprinkle of Chili Powder
1/8 tsp coriander, ground
¼ tsp Korintje cinnamon
¼ tsp Himalaya pink salt
1 tsp (heaping) garbanzo bean *miso* mixed with 3 tsp soup broth

Place water, squash, onion, celery, chili powder, coriander, cinnamon, and salt into a soup pot with a lid
Cook with lid on medium heat about 20 minutes
Using a manual potato masher, mash the soup in the pot being careful not to splash hot soup
Try to get all the squash pieces mashed as finely as possible

Cook another 5 minutes on medium heat with lid on
Turn off heat and add miso mixture, blending well
Let cool for about 15 minutes
Transfer soup into a blender cup and process soup until creamy about 35 seconds

Reheat soup, but don't boil it, as boiling changes the taste and miso nutrient value

Garbanzo Bean Miso Soup
1 liter water
1 onion, chopped
3 ribs celery, chopped
2 Tbsp. Braggs Amino Acids
Place all ingredients into a soup pot; bring to a boil for 3 minutes.

Add:
1 15 oz. can garbanzo beans, drained—not rinsed
3 Tbsp. fresh cilantro, chopped
1 tsp. turmeric
Zest of 1 lemon (lemon rind)
Cook on medium heat for 20 minutes and then remove from heat

Add:
2 tsp garbanzo bean miso with enough soup broth to make a thin paste
Mix well and serve

Quick Fresh Vegetable Broth for Cooking Grains or as Consommé
2 cups water
½ small carrot, grated
½ inch fresh ginger, peeled and cut into 3 pieces

1 large garlic clove, cut into slices
1 tsp Braggs Amino Acids
Place all ingredients into a saucepan; bring to a boil and simmer for 5 minutes.
Strain and use broth to cook grains or as consommé

Buckwheat Groats cooked in Vegetable Broth [Gluten-free]
To the above Vegetable Broth recipe after its been strained

Add:
¼ cup dry buckwheat groats [gluten-free despite its name]
½ cup water
Cook on medium heat about 8 minutes until tender
This makes a nice substitute for pasta, potatoes, or rice.

Catherine's Ultimate Vegetable Soup
This recipe makes about 18 soup ladles of wonderful chorba-style soup. All vegetables should be chopped bite size. You can portion-pack and freeze some.

1 ½ quarts or liters water
1 cup green cabbage, chopped
1 sweet onion, chopped
1 leek, chopped
4 ribs celery, chopped
2 carrots, chopped
1 medium potato, chopped into small pieces
½ cup fresh green beans, chopped
½ cup fresh wax beans, chopped
2/3 cup frozen lima beans
2/3 cup frozen green peas

½ tsp Himalaya pink salt
Pinch or two of cayenne pepper
½ tsp dill weed
1 ½ cups canned whole tomatoes, mashed (I use only glass jar imported Italian organic tomatoes)

Into a large soup pot with a lid, place the water and add vegetables as you chop them
Once the water has come to a boil, turn it down to medium low
After all the veggies are in the pot, put the lid on and turn the heat/fire down to low (No. 2 on electric range) and cook for 30 minutes with lid on
Vegetables will be *a la dente* and contain many enzymes due to low heat cooking. That's the key to nutrition in soup vegetables: low heat cooking and *a la dente!*

Add:
½ cup fresh parsley, chopped
1 bunch scallions, chopped
Mix well into hot soup, as they will be blanched from the soup heat.
Don't boil soup when reheating.

Vegetable Miso Soup
Use the above recipe *but do not include* potatoes, tomatoes, dill weed, and parsley.
You can substitute 2/3 cup butternut squash cubes.
After 30 minutes of cooking with lid on the pot, turn off the heat and

Add:
1 Tbsp. garbanzo miso [gluten-free] mixed with 3 Tbsp. soup broth to make a thin paste
Mix well into vegetable soup and serve

Do not boil when reheating soup.

Oriental-style Vegetable Miso Soup
1 ½ quarts or liters water
¾ cup green cabbage, sliced thin
2 carrots, thinly sliced
½ onion, thinly sliced
3 ribs Bok Choy (not Baby Bok Choy), small dice and use leaves
2 cloves garlic, chopped
1 Tbsp. fresh ginger, chopped small
6 Shiitake mushrooms, stems removed and thinly sliced
12 fresh snow peas, ends and strings removed
2 Tbsp. Braggs Amino Acids

Place all ingredients into a large soup pot; bring to a boil; turn heat to medium and cook for 15 minutes

Add:
1 cup baby spinach leaves
4 oz. firm tofu, small dice
Cook for on medium low heat for 3 minutes.
Remove from heat

Add:
1 Tbsp. garbanzo miso mixed with 2 Tbsp. soup broth to make a thin paste
Mix well into soup

Add:
1 bunch scallions, thinly sliced
To reheat, don't boil.

Note: This soup recipe also can be made without the miso paste.

Broccoli-Cauliflower Miso Soup

1 quart or liter water
2 ½ cups broccoli, chopped
2/3 cup cauliflower, chopped
1/3 cup fennel, thinly sliced
½ cup sweet onion, chopped
½ cup celery, chopped
1 small potato, thinly sliced
¼ tsp Himalaya pink salt
½ tsp dill weed

Place all ingredients into a soup pot with a lid; bring to a boil; turn down heat to medium and cook 35 minutes with the lid on the pot
Turn off heat and using a potato masher, mash soup to make a thick consistency
Be careful not to splash hot soup

Add:
1 heaping tsp garbanzo bean miso mixed with 2 Tbsp. soup liquid to make a thin paste
Mix thoroughly
When reheating, don't boil soup.
After soup is cooled, you can process it in a blender to make a "cream" style soup.
This soup is even tastier the next day!

Crème Soups Using NO Dairy and Gluten-free

Crème of Asparagus

1 quart or liter water, boiling
2 Tbsp. EV olive oil

1 ½ lbs. green asparagus, cleaned and chopped
3 ribs celery, chopped
1 large sweet onion, chopped
1 small potato, peeled and grated on the large hole of a grater
½ tsp dried dill weed
½ tsp Himalaya pink salt
Pinch or two cayenne powder

Heat the oil in a large soup pot, which has a lid
Add onions, celery, asparagus—in that order—potato, salt, pepper, and dill weed
Sauté and mix well on medium heat so as not to scorch or burn veggies
Keep mixing until water comes to a boil, or at least 3 minutes
Add boiling water to veggies, turn down heat to low (1 ½ on electric stove)
Cover pot with lid and cook for 40 minutes
Check occasionally to adjust for salt and pepper taste
When cooked, allow to cool for at least 30 minutes off heat

To cream
Using a blender, place enough soup to fill a blender cup half way.
Process the soup at least 1 minute. Process the remaining soup the same way.
Serve Cream of Asparagus soup either hot or cold.

Note: the nutritional benefits of asparagus are that it's a great food source of glutathione, one of the prime detoxifying antioxidants and helps people with any type of kidney ailments.

Crème of Broccoli
Use the above recipe and method only substitute
3 cups broccoli, chopped, for the asparagus

Optional: 1 garlic clove, chopped

Crème of Carrot
Use the above recipe and method only substitute
3 cups carrots, chopped, for the asparagus
No potato; instead add ¼ cup fresh fennel, thinly sliced from the bulb end
1 tsp fresh ginger, peeled and grated
No dill weed; instead add ¼ tsp of Korintje cinnamon OR 1/8 tsp nutmeg

Crème of Cauliflower
Use the above recipe and method only substitute
3 cups cauliflower, chopped, for the asparagus

Crème of Zucchini
Use the above recipe and method only substitute
3 medium-size zucchini, chopped, for the asparagus

Soup for Breakfast
One of the most filling breakfasts that I enjoy is to heat one of the crème soups (2 or 3 ladlesful) to which I add 3 to 4 heaping tablespoonful of cooked quinoa. It certainly is tasty, sticks with me for a long time, and definitely is much more nutritious than any pour-out-of-the-box, sugar-coated, ersatz fruity tasting cereal with low fat or skim milk, in my opinion.

Healthful Snacks – When You Are Ready for Them

*D*oes it mean that to maintain vibrant health you won't be able to eat treats or snacks? Not necessarily! However, the more healthful and balanced a daily diet you maintain, the less likely it is that you will be reaching for snacks of any type—healthful or junk.

Once you and your body chemistry realize that *proper whole foods nutrition* is being provided regularly, most—if not all—symptomology starts to diminish to the point where, eventually, all cravings become non-existent. You slim down; have more energy; face and skin clear up; no more aches, pains, intestinal problems, GERD (Gastrointestinal Reflux Disease), high blood pressure, etc. How does that sound?

Just to let you know that I think I know what I'm talking about, may I tell you something of my story? I'm 78 years old; weigh 123 pounds—the same as when I was 25 years old; don't eat snacks often and never junk food; eat three nutritious and balanced meals a day based in plant foods—maybe once in a blue moon I'll eat an organic egg omelet for Sunday brunch at an organic Bistro; have two to three fully-formed foot-long bowel movements every day; and my blood pressure reading is 110/62! And, I take NO prescription medications! What am I doing wrong? Or, should I ask, what have I been doing right? If you've been reading this book, you probably can figure out: I practice what I preach or as some would say, "I walk the talk."

I share that personal information because at one time I was almost dead—literally—due to having been mistreated medically by the irresponsible prescribing of pharmaceutical drugs. The drugs were killing me, the more they were giving me, the more I couldn't function. I guess I was like many of you probably are feeling, but a lot worse. I even had a "near death experience" that was the best thing that ever happened to me.

That experience changed my life. I realized that there were other healthcare modalities that did not poison a body into wellness with pharmaceuticals which, in many instances, are questionable as to real efficacy. I went back to school; matriculated in *natural nutrition and holistic health sciences*; and learned back in the 1970s and '80s what *real, holistic* nutrition for the body is, and what researchers have started to publish only in the last several years. I vividly remember in the 1980s a medical doctor challenging me with this statement: "If there was something to nutrition, don't you think we [medicine] would know about it?" Oh, the disillusionments some people live with!

The only time I shop for, or use, snacking foods is when I am traveling. I reason that healthful, organic snacks, which pack easily in my brief case, suit case, or car, are much better for me than anything I can buy while on the road or in a fast food place, plus are GMO-free too! What do I take with me?

First, let me tell you what I don't pack: Any chips, munchies, etc., cooked, fried, or baked using oils. They always seem rancid, in my opinion, because of all the high heat involved in production. When one opens the bag, one can smell that rancid "fried oil" odor that, to me, is indicative of heat damage from cooking oil, I contend, including starchy carbohydrates damage in the form of acrylamides[252].

The other thing I don't pack is protein bars, as too many of them contain many ingredients that I don't approve of because of their digestibility challenges, e.g., agave[253], coconut oil,[254] and protein powders from questionable sources that may contain heavy metals[255], i.e., arsenic in rice, or GMO ingredients.

Online there's a review of protein bars, "The Best and Worst: Protein and Nutrition Bars"[256], which you may be interested in reading while also keeping in mind my comments.

I include in my travel snack pack fresh organic fruits like apples, oranges, and a couple organic baby bananas; organic rice cake for breakfast, if I can't find a suitable grain; *Lara Bars,* which are made with dried dates, other dried fruits, and nuts; maybe a *GoMacro Macrobar;* or *Two Moms Raw Nut Bar*—Blueberry Burst is my favorite; and my favorite snack—seaweed in individual small packets: *GimMe Organic Roasted Sesame Snacks* or *Chipotle SeaSnax,* which satisfy any salty taste desire I may have instead of eating chips. Plus seaweed provides loads of trace minerals. For folks who are concerned about gluten, *Larabar* has a relatively new product, *"Larabar Uber Crunchy Nut Bar,"* which contains

---

252 http://www.fda.gov/Food/FoodborneIllnessContaminants/ChemicalContaminants/ucm053569.htm accessed 3-22-16
253 http://articles.mercola.com/sites/articles/archive/2010/03/30/beware-of-the-agave-nectar-health-food.aspx accessed 1-21-16
254 http://www.livestrong.com/article/141282-bad-effects-using-coconut-oil/ accessed 1-21-16
255 http://www.naturalnews.com/045108_vegan_proteins_heavy_metals_laboratory_test_results.html accessed 1-21-16
256 http://www.theholykale.com/2013/08/the-best-and-worst-protein-and-nutrition-bars/ accessed 1-21-16

almonds, dates, brown rice syrup, toasted coconut, Macadamia nuts, cashews, honey, and sea salt—all Non-GMO, gluten-free, and kosher!

All those snacks will see me through any trip, and I usually return home with a few uneaten. The other all-important thing I pack is my bottled-in-glass water. Won't leave home without it! I carry small glass bottles of alkaline-base water to take with me to meetings, etc., plus liter-size glass bottles in my car for my hotel room. No chocolate, potato chips, or candy bars; all wholesome, organic food!

Do my snacks sound weird? Maybe they do now, but once you start eating to beat disease, I think you probably will find yourself choosing some of them too.

Quick Tips for Healthful Eating

Tip No. 1
Purchase, prepare/cook, and eat foods that are NOT genetically modified or grown (GM, GMO). Instead, choose organically- and sustainably-grown plant-based and animal-source foods.

Tip No. 2
Eliminate all food processing chemicals, artificial ingredients, colors, and iodized salt from your diet and foods. For salt, use Himalayan pink salt or clean sea salt from waters not affected by Fukushima.

Tip No. 3
No artificial sugars of any kind and reduce cane sugar consumption dramatically, if not totally.

Tip No. 4
Drink and cook with non-fluoridated, non-chloraminated water. If need be, install a reverse osmosis under-the-kitchen-sink water

filter[257] so that the water you drink and cook with is as chemical-free as possible.

Tip No. 5
Do not fry any animal or plant-based foods. Be very careful about the oil you use for preparing food. Polyunsaturated oils and partially hydrogenated fats are not healthful oils, I offer.

Tip No. 6
Daily eat 50 percent of your diet as raw, unprocessed whole foods such as salads, fruits, nuts, fermented veggies, sprouts, and fresh-pressed vegetable juices.

One of the best raw food resources for exquisitely prepared raw, plant-based (vegan) *gourmet quality* food is the book *Conscious Eating* available on Amazon.com at
http://www.amazon.com/Conscious-Eating-Gabriel-Cousens-M-D/dp/1556432852.

Vegetarian Travel Guide Information
Every state and large USA metropolitan areas
http://www.vegetarianusa.com/index.html

Vegetarian Bed & Breakfasts
Every state in the USA
http://www.vegetarianusa.com/vegetarianbedbreakfast.html

Vegetarian Vacations (24 Countries)
http://www.vegetarianusa.com/vacationmapworld2000.html

---

257 http://bestreviews.com/best-water-filter-systems

Wellness Vacation
http://treeoflifecenterus.com/category/tr_programs/wellness_vacation/

Health Rejuvenations Center and Resort
Dr. Gabriel Cousens Tree of Life Center (Patagonia, Arizona)
http://treeoflifecenterus.com/

How to Expand Your Knowledge about Nutrition, Health, and Healing

Ever since I almost died in my early thirties as a result of medical mistakes, I've become an ardent student, practitioner, researcher, author, devotee—plus voracious reader—of information regarding issues that affect human health—especially the seedy "politics of health"—since I've learned that there is more out there that vested interests don't want the average person to know about, and there's much controlled media hype to keep it that way, in my opinion.

Knowledge is power, and you eventually become an independent thinker when you know more—especially scientific facts and published research—just not hype and public relations spin intended to steer consumers toward certain vested-interests' agendas and proselytizing memes.

I encourage everyone to expand your knowledge base and read books that will open doors and pathways to understanding how to take care of your health and body so that you age gracefully; don't have to take four or more prescription medications every day; and you can enjoy life to its fullest without pain or dis-ease.

As an aside, may I state again that I'm 78 years old, and everyone tells me that I look like I'm in my 50s? It's truly amusing to see mouths drop open in surprise when people find out my actual age. My standard remark is that it's either true or my birth certificate lies.

Some books, which I think will help you understand more about and how to "eat to beat disease," plus maintain *optimum health*, are:

- *Altered Genes, Twisted Truth*
  Steven M. Druker / Clear River Press / ISBN-13: 978-0-9856169-0-8
    "How the Venture to Genetically Engineer Our Food Has Subverted Science, Corrupted Government, and Systematically Deceived the Public"
- *The Disease Delusion*
  Jeffrey S Bland, PhD / Harper Wave / ISBN 978-0-06-229073-1
    "Conquering the Causes of Chronic Illness for a Healthier, Longer, and Happier Life"
- *Eat Fat, Get Thin: Why the Fat We Eat Is the Key to Sustained Weight Loss and Vibrant Health*
    Mark Hyman, MD / Little, Brown and Company / ISBN 978-0-316-33883-7
- *Food Forensics, The Health Ranger's Guide to Foods that Harm and Foods that Heal*
    Mike Adams / BenBella Books / 2016 / Amazon.com
- *How Not to Die: Discover the Foods Scientifically Proven to Prevent and Reverse Disease* Michael Greger, MD with Gene Stone / Flatiron Books-Macmillan Corp. /
    ISBN 978-1-250-06611-4 / 2015 / *The New York Times Best Seller list*
- *The Juice Lady's Guide to Juicing for Health*
  Cherie Calbom, MS / Avery / ISBN 978-1-58333-317-4

"A practical A-to-Z guide to the prevention and treatment of the most common health disorders"
- *Natural Healing Encyclopedia*
  Mark Stengler, NMD (licensed naturopathic doctor, San Diego, CA)
  Publisher: Health Revelations (www.healthrevelations.com) 702 Cathedral Street, Baltimore, MD 21201 / 2015

Newsletters Online—all are holistic-complementary-medicine oriented

- *Tree of Life Newsletter,* Gabriel Cousens, MD
- *Healing Newsletter,* The Gerson Institute
- Joseph Mercola, DO, *Mercola.com, The World's #1 Natural Health Website*
- *Self Healing,* a newsletter by Andrew Weil, MD

Filing Consumer Complaints about Food Products

If consumers have complaints about FDA-regulated food products, the U.S. Food and Drug Administration offer online a resource for registering complaints. "Consumer Complaint Coordinators" are available via telephones in each state to take consumers phone calls.

The listing includes information for all 50 states, the District of Columbia, Puerto Rico, and the U.S. Virgin Islands

http://www.fda.gov/Safety/ReportaProblem/ConsumerComplaintCoordinators/default.htm

Recipes from Catherine's Kitchen

All ingredients ought to be organically grown and non-GMO.

Caramelized Butternut Squash
2 heaping cups butternut squash, cubed or a 20 oz. packaged precut fresh butternut squash
1 Tbsp. (scant) EV olive oil
Sprinkling of Himalaya pink salt
½ tsp Korintje cinnamon
Sprinkling of ground cardamom
Cayenne pepper to taste

Using a little olive oil, grease the sides and bottom of a 9 inch glass pie pan
Add squash; drizzle olive oil; mix to coat all pieces
Sprinkle salt, cinnamon, cardamom, and pepper; mix again
Bake in a 375° oven uncovered for 1 hour or a little longer until soft
Mix every 20 minutes
Squash becomes caramelized a little

Baked Cabbage Casserole

¼ head medium size green cabbage, core removed and sliced thin
1 small red potato cut in half, then cut into thin slices
4 Cremini or Baby Bella mushrooms, sliced thin
1/8 tsp Himalaya pink salt
Pinch or two of cayenne pepper
¼ tsp dried dill weed

Use an oven proof casserole. Grease sides and bottom with some olive oil placed on a paper towel.
Place all ingredients into the casserole and mix well.
Add 1 tsp EV olive oil and mix well to coat everything.
Sprinkle 2 Tbsp. water on top.
Place tin foil over top the casserole.
Bake in 375° oven 35-45 minutes. Mix at 20 minutes.

Lemon Roasted Carrots

6 carrots peeled and cut into diagonal pieces 1/8 inch thick
2 medium lemons juiced
Zest of 1 lemon
2 tsp EV olive oil
Himalaya pink salt and cayenne pepper to taste
½ cup parsley chopped

Place all ingredients except parsley into a large bowl; mix very well
Transfer bowl contents to lasagna baking pan or large cookie sheet
Spread carrots evenly
Bake in a 375° oven 45-50 minutes until carrots are *a la dente* – not cooked soft
Remove from oven and allow cooling for 15 minutes

Transfer to a bowl; add parsley and mix to coat all carrots
Serve warm or as a cold veggie side dish

Sicilian Cauliflower
Cauliflower should be cooked in a vegetable steamer and allowed to cool before proceeding with finishing the recipe.

6 cauliflower florets broken into same size smaller florets
6 fresh garlic cloves, peeled
Juice of 1 lemon diluted with 2 Tbsp. water
1 Tbsp. EV olive oil
¼ tsp Himalaya pink salt
Red pepper flakes (Pepperoncini) to taste
2 Tbsp. fresh parsley, chopped
Parmesan Reggiano cheese flakes (optional)

Cook cauliflower and garlic cloves in a vegetable steamer until *a la dente*. Drink the left over cooking water as there are plenty of nutrients, especially the mineral molybdenum.
Allow cooling completely, especially if using cheese, which would melt—you want cheese flakes
Cut garlic cloves in half and place into a bowl with cauliflower
Combine lemon juice, water, olive oil and salt; mix well
Drizzle over veggies; add cheese, pepper flakes, and parsley; mix well
Enjoy as a cold Italian-style antipasto vegetable

"Confetti" Corn (if you like corn, you'll love this recipe) (Gluten-free)
2 Tbsp. EV olive oil
2 small shallots, minced

¼ sweet red pepper, chopped small
¼ sweet orange pepper, chopped small
¼ sweet green pepper, chopped small
1 heaping cup frozen ORGANIC corn *only* as most corn is GMO; or freshly shucked off the cob in summer
¼ tsp organic Chili Powder
1/8 tsp Himalayan pink salt
½ fresh lime, juiced (more, if you like lime)

Heat olive oil in a 10 inch stainless steel skillet
Add shallots and peppers. Sauté on medium heat for 2 to 3 minutes, mixing often
Add corn, chili powder, salt, and lime juice
Cook on medium heat, stirring often, until corn is cooked thru and hot, about 2-3 minutes

---

Cucumber Salad

½ organic English cucumber, skin scrubbed well, not peeled, chopped coarsely
¼ sweet onion, finely diced
¼ cup fresh parsley, chopped
10 cherry tomatoes cut in half or quarters
1 inner yellow rib of celery, diced
1 lemon juiced
3 Tbsp. water
1 tsp honey
¼ tsp Himalaya pink salt
Pinch or two of cayenne pepper

Place cucumber, onion, parsley, tomatoes, and celery into a bowl
In a separate bowl, mix lemon juice and honey until honey dissolves; add water, salt, and pepper

A stick infusion blender could be used to mix the dressing
Pour dressing over veggies and mix well
Refrigerate for at least 1 hr before serving

Szechuan Style Green Beans (Gluten-free, mildly spicy)
½ lb. fresh green beans cleaned and cut in half
2 shallots, minced
8 Shiitake mushrooms, stems removed and chopped coarsely
2 Tbsp. fresh ginger, minced
2 cloves garlic, minced
1/8 to ¼ tsp dried red pepper flakes (Pepperoncini) depending upon your taste for heat
1 Tbsp. Braggs Amino Acids
2 Tbsp. water
½ tsp toasted sesame oil
2 Tbsp. EV olive oil

Heat olive oil in a 10 inch stainless steel fry pan
Add green beans, shallots, mushrooms, ginger, and red pepper flakes
Turn heat to medium and sauté veggies for 5 minutes
Add Braggs Amino Acids and water
Cover fry pan with a lid or tin foil; turn heat to medium low and steam veggies for 3-5 minutes
String beans should be *a la dente*
Turn off heat; add sesame oil; mix well
Garnish optional: 1 Tbsp. toasted sesame seeds

Serve hot or cold

The NO Pasta, Pasta—Italian Style (Gluten-free)

3 medium size zucchini, cut with a julienne peeler, spiralizer (or mandolin--be careful of fingers!)
Or a mixture/medley of 2 zucchini and 1 yellow squash
1 cup Cremini mushrooms, sliced
2 small onions, sliced (there's slightly different tastes when using either red, sweet, or yellow onions; I prefer sweet white onions or Vidalia onions)
1 cup chopped fresh ripe tomato
2 tsp garlic, minced
1/8 tsp dry pepper flakes (Pepperoncini)
3 Tbsp. EV olive oil (1 Tbsp. for preparing squash pasta; 2 Tbsp. for sauce)
¼ tsp Himalaya pink salt

Squash 'Pasta'
Two ways to prepare it:
No. 1: Steam squash pasta in a vegetable steamer until just *a la dente*. Cover with lid and keep warm until sauce is ready.
No. 2: Sauté zucchini in 1 Tbsp. EV olive oil until just tender. Set aside and keep warm to make sauce.

Sauce
In a separate fry pan, heat 2 Tbsp. EV olive oil
Add mushrooms, onions, garlic, red pepper flakes, and sauté on medium heat for 2 to 3 minutes
Add tomatoes and salt
Sauté another 3 to 4 minutes using medium-low heat
Mix well

To plate:
Place zucchini pasta on a large plate or in a pasta bowl and top with vegetable sauce.

Optional: Garnish with 2 Tbsp. chopped parsley and *Parmigiana Reggiano* cheese shavings, if you eat cheese.

Potatoes Unlike You've Eaten Before: Vegan, low fat, and uniquely delicious!

Different Mashed Potatoes

Depending upon how you like mashed potatoes, you either can peel them or leave their skins on for more nutritional value. However, if you leave the skins on, make certain to scrub them thoroughly and to cut out any dark or suberized spots.

3 red potatoes cut into small chunks
Water to cover potatoes in the pot
3-4 Tbsp. lite coconut milk
Himalaya pink salt
Cayenne pepper to taste

Place potatoes into a pot covered with water; bring to a boil and cook until soft
Drain potatoes leaving a tiny residue of cook water
Mash potatoes using a hand-held potato masher
Add coconut milk, salt, and pepper
Mash until thick and creamy, adding a tad bit of coconut milk if needed

Variation No. 2

To the above recipe add
½ cup frozen peas, cooked and drained
Mix well without mashing the peas

Variation No. 3
To the above two recipes add
1/8 tsp curry powder
These mashed potatoes taste like the inside of an Indian cuisine samosa.

Baked Potato
Since a potato is high on the Glycemic List, I suggest eating smaller size potatoes rather than standard huge size baking potatoes. Personally, I think red potatoes have the best texture and taste.
After the potato has been baked, instead of dressing it with butter, sour cream, or cheese, try this for an exceptional taste treat: Add ¼ to ½ ripe avocado at room temperature mixed into the potato with salt and pepper. I think you will enjoy it tremendously.

Red Beet Salad
4 red beets of the same size, tops and tails removed, scrubbed thoroughly

Place prepared red beets onto the middle rung of a toaster oven on aluminum foil to prevent red beet juice from ruining the oven.

Dressing
½ lemon, juiced
1 tsp EV olive oil
¼ tsp Himalaya pink salt
Pinch or two of cayenne pepper
Mix well to blend.

Bake at 400° for 1 hr 15 mins for medium size beets or up to 1 hr 30 mins for larger beets

Remove from oven and allow cooling to peel skin without burning your fingers
Cut beets in half, then half again, and cut each piece in half, making chunks
Place beet chunks into a bowl
Add dressing and mix well
Refrigerate for at least 1 hour

Serving suggestion:

- Side vegetable dish
- Mixed greens salad topping
- Condiment

Oven Roasted Vegetable Entrée

This recipe uses a large oven-proof pan—something like a huge, deep quiche pan or lasagna pan. This makes a lot of vegetables and is good for a dinner party, or 3 or 4 reheated dinners.

20 small Brussel sprouts cleaned and bottom stem section cut off
1 large sweet red pepper, cut into chunks
2 carrots cut into coins
1 potato, skin on, cut into medium chunks
1 small zucchini cut into ¾ inch coins
10 thick asparagus spears cut into thirds
1 large sweet onion, large chop
OR 12 small pearl-size red or white onions, peeled and left whole
1 small yam cut into coins
4 cloves garlic, minced
2 Tbsp. or more, fresh thyme leaves
1 lemon juiced

2 Tbsp. EV olive oil
Himalaya pink salt and cayenne pepper to taste

Lightly oil the sides and bottom of an oven-proof pan.
As you prep veggies, place them into the pan starting with Brussel sprouts. Bury asparagus inside the mixture so they don't cook to a crisp and dry out.
Make certain to end with onions, garlic, and thyme leaves on top.
Drizzle lemon juice and olive oil all over the top of the veggies.
Add salt and pepper to taste.
Mix well.
Bake uncovered in a 375° oven 1 hr 15 mins to 1 hr 30 mins, depending when the potatoes are cooked.
Mix every 20 minutes.

Serving suggestion:
The recipe can be cut in half to make a smaller size entrée.
If not used as an entrée or vegetable dish for several diners, portion veggies into oven-proof individual-size baking ramekins, cover with plastic wrap and refrigerate to reheat as lunch or dinner for a couple of days.

- Mixed green salad with watercress and cherry tomatoes
- Side of fermented vegetables or
- Cup of soup, preferably a bean soup

Ramen Noodles with Asian-style Stir-fry Vegetables (Gluten-free)

Ramen Noodles
1 cake [4 cakes to a package] of *Lotus Foods Organic Millet & Brown Rice Ramen Noodles* (2.5 oz. dry weight) cooked according to package

directions and drained well. Time the cooking for the noodles so they are ready when the stir-fry is done.

Hint: Prepare all veggies and as you prep, place them in a salad bowl so as to have them ready to go into the stir fry pan as called for in the recipe timing. Layer them so that the Bok Choy and spinach are on the bottom of the bowl and then add peppers, mushrooms, and onions. That way when you empty the bowl into the pan, veggies needing more time and heat before stirring are first in the pan.

Stir-fry Vegetables
2 Tbsp. EV olive oil
8 Shiitake mushrooms, stems removed, and cut into ribbons
1 medium sweet onion, chopped
1 cup total mixture of red, yellow, and orange sweet peppers, chopped
1 cup Bok Choy, chopped, (not baby Bok Choy) use green leaves too
½ cup baby spinach leaves
2 cloves garlic, minced
½ inch of fresh ginger, peeled and minced
¼ lb. extra firm tofu, drained and cubed small (optional)
2 Tbsp. Braggs Amino Acids
¾ tsp toasted Sesame oil
1 tsp peanut butter
2 Tbsp. water
½ tsp honey

Garnish
2 Tbsp. fresh cilantro, chopped
2 Tbsp. dry roasted peanuts, chopped (optional)
4 scallions, thinly sliced

Heat oil and sauté mushrooms, onion, peppers, and Bok Choy on medium heat 3 to 5 minutes
Add spinach, garlic, and ginger
Mix Braggs, sesame oil, peanut butter, water, and honey together to make a smooth sauce that you add to the veggies
Sauté on medium heat 2 minutes
Add tofu; stir and cook until tofu is heated through
Plate drained warm ramen noodles into a large serving dish to make a bed for the stir fry
Pour stir fry over ramen noodles
Garnish with cilantro, peanuts, and scallions

Chinese Style Stir Fry (Gluten-free)
Hint: prepare all the vegetables and place them into a large bowl or colander as you prep so that you can place all veggies into the fry pan or wok at the same time. Cooking time is very short and veggies are *a la dent*.

2 Tbsp. EV olive oil
½ cup onion, chopped
6 Shiitake mushrooms, stems removed and chopped
1 carrot, chopped
3 broccoli florets broken into smaller florets
2 ribs Bok Choy (not baby Bok Choy) use leaves too, chopped
Handful snow peas, ends and strings removed
2 cloves garlic, chopped
1 Tbsp. ginger, chopped
¼ tsp red pepper flakes (Pepperoncini)
1 Tbsp. Braggs Amino Acids
½ tsp toasted sesame oil

Optional: ¼ lb. firm tofu cubes
Garnish: Sliced scallions and toasted sesame seeds

Heat oil in a 10 inch stainless steel fry pan or in a large wok
Add all prepped vegetables
Turn heat to medium and stir constantly to coat all veggies with oil to keep from sticking
Turn heat down to medium and stir fry for about 5 minutes
Add pepper flakes, Braggs, sesame oil, and tofu cubes; continue stir frying for 2 or 3 minutes
Garnish with scallion slices and toasted sesame seeds

Serving suggestion:

- For a Chinese style meal, start off with Mushroom Miso Soup, and then enjoy Chinese style stir fry with a serving of brown or mixed rice, and Szechuan Style Green Beans. Top it off with Green tea or my favorite, Jasmine Green tea.

Hijiki Sea Weed Salad
Before starting this recipe, soak Hijiki sea weed in enough water to cover so that it can be ready to use when you have the rest of this recipe set.

4 Tbsp. dry Hijiki sea weed, soaked
½ cup carrots, slivered or grated
½ sweet onion, sliced into thin moons
½ cup fresh green beans, julienned
1 tsp organic safflower oil
1 ½ tsp Braggs Amino Acids
1 tsp honey

1 tsp fresh ginger, grated finely
Pinch or two of cayenne pepper
1 tsp toasted sesame oil

Heat safflower oil in a 10 inch stainless steel fry pan
Add carrots, onions, and green beans stirring constantly over medium heat for 3-4 minutes
Drain sea weed and add to veggies
Add Braggs Amino Acids, honey, ginger, and pepper
Simmer 5 minutes over medium heat, mixing often
Remove from heat and add sesame oil; mix well
Refrigerate and serve cold

Fresh Tomato Salad

1 ripe tomato (Heirlooms are the best!) at room temperature sliced into thick "steaks"
2 Tbsp. fresh parsley chopped
¼ lemon, juiced
½ tsp olive oil
Himalaya pink salt and cayenne pepper to taste

Arrange tomato slices on a plate; sprinkle salt and pepper, then parsley
Combine lemon juice and olive oil then drizzle over tomato steaks
Allow salad to sit at room temperature for at least 5 minutes for flavors to marinate

Serving suggestion:

- As a side vegetable
- On top of a bed of mix greens

- As a topping for an open face sandwich made with guacamole or sliced avocado (or hummus) and sprouts, if you can eat sprouted whole grain bread.

    Build an open face sandwich: Slice of bread, sliced avocado, grated cheese if you eat dairy, finely chopped red onion, sprouts, marinated tomato slices; or you can make a wrap using the same ingredients.

Veggie Sauté
Prep all veggies, placing them into a bowl, until all are ready for the pan. The cooking part moves fast.

2 Tbsp. EV olive oil
½ onion, chopped large
½ medium zucchini, julienned
6 mushrooms, quartered
½ cup celeriac root, julienned
1 Tbsp. fresh ginger, peeled and minced
3 broccoli florets broken smaller
8 snow peas, ends and strings removed
2 cloves garlic, chopped
¼ tsp red pepper flakes
2 Tbsp. Braggs Amino Acids
¼ lb. firm tofu, cubed
4 scallions, sliced

Heat olive oil in a 10 inch stainless steel fry pan
Add all veggies and red peppers flakes; stir constantly for about 7 minutes on medium heat
Add Braggs Amino Acids and tofu; cook on medium heat until tofu is heated
Garnish with scallions

Serving suggestion:

- Side of cooked brown or wild rice or quinoa
- Tossed mixed green salad with lemon juice and olive oil dressing
- Side of fermented beets

Sweet Treats

Chia Seed Pudding
1/3 cup organic chia seeds, rinsed very well and drained
1 15 oz. can organic coconut milk-lite
1 Tbsp. mild honey (alfalfa, clover, or orange)
½ tsp organic vanilla

Combine all ingredients in a fair size mixing bowl; mix very well at least an hour before serving time to allow it to 'jell'. Refrigerate.

Serving Suggestions:
Chia Seed Pudding can be served with fresh berries or sliced banana as garnishes.
It can be eaten as part of a fruit breakfast or a snack treat.
It can be eaten as dessert after any meal, but don't garnish with fresh fruit, as that would not be a proper food combination for healthful digestive integrity after eating a meal.

Chia Nutrition Information
2 times the potassium of bananas
2 times the protein of other seeds or grains
2 times the fiber in a cup of oatmeal
3 times the iron in spinach
3 times the antioxidant potency of blueberries

5 times the calcium in milk

2 Tablespoons of chia seeds contain 4 grams of protein and 8.3 grams of fiber.

Additional ways to use chia seeds:
Sprinkle on salads for crunch
Add to homemade salad dressings
Add to smoothies
A substitute for poppy seeds
Enrich breakfast cereals with them
Use as toppings for ice cream, puddings, and custards

The No-Egg, Egg Nog (a great holiday drink) (Gluten-free)
1 cup filtered water
1 cup almond milk (homemade preferred)
1 cup unsalted cashews (soaked at least for 30 minutes)
½ cup unsalted macadamia nuts (soaked at least for 30 minutes)
3 dates, pitted OR 2 Tbsp. organic maple syrup, B grade
1 tsp vanilla
½ tsp ground Korintje cinnamon
½ tsp ground nutmeg
Pinch of Himalaya pink salt

Soak cashews and macadamia nuts in filtered water for at least 30 minutes, and drain well.
Discard soak water.
Combine all ingredients into a blender cup and blend very well until thick and smooth.
If too thick, add a little more almond milk and blend well.

Serve chilled.
Optional: Garnish with a slight dusting of Korintje cinnamon or nutmeg
Serves 6-8

Hat tip to and adapted from Nutrition Stripped / McKel Hill, MS, RD, LDN
http://nutritionstripped.com/egg-not-nog/

Homemade Raw Almond Milk (Gluten-free)
1 cup of raw whole almonds (unpasteurized preferred)
4-6 cups of filtered water
1 tsp vanilla or 1 vanilla bean
2 Tbsp. raw honey (a tad more if you like it sweeter)

Soak almonds overnight, plus the vanilla bean if using that, in enough water to cover generously.
Discard soak water and rinse almonds and vanilla bean.
Place almonds, vanilla bean chopped, and honey into a blender cup along with filtered water.
Start with 4 cups of water as you may want to thin it out a little, if too thick.
When processed to thickness desired, pour almond mixture into a cheese cloth or mesh nut bag. Squeeze the almond mixture in the cloth/bag as dry as you can squeeze it into a large bowl.
The final step is to pour the almond milk through a fine sieve to catch any 'crumbs' that may be left.
This will keep 5 to 6 days in the refrigerator.

Note: This homemade almond milk is so much more delicious, I think, and definitely more healthful than commercial almond milks, which can contain ingredients such as Gellan Gum (an exopolysaccharide created by bacterial fermentation), Carrageenan (which can cause digestive issues), Potassium Citrate (can cause diarrhea, vomiting, nausea and stomach pain), Sunflower Lecithin, Natural Flavors (could include GMOs or chemicals), Calcium carbonate (chalk; an antacid that can cause constipation).

The left-over almond pulp can be used to make cookies or a pie crust. Hat tip to and adapted from Tasty Yummies recipes

Pumpkin Custard Pudding
This tastes better than pumpkin pie and is baked in individual custard cups. My dinner guests always look forward to this as their dessert.

1 15 oz. can of organic pumpkin
½ tsp organic Pumpkin Pie spice mix
½ tsp Korintje cinnamon
2 pinches of Himalaya pink salt
1 cup organic lite coconut milk
2 Tbsp. mild honey (acacia, clover, or orange)
1 tsp organic vanilla
2 organic, free-range eggs, beaten

Into a large bowl, place pumpkin, spice mix, cinnamon, and salt; mix very well and set aside
In another bowl, combine coconut milk, honey, and vanilla; mix well to dissolve the honey
Add the liquid mixture to the pumpkin mixture
Add beaten eggs to the pumpkin mixture; mix very well
Ladle into 6 individual custard cups
Bake in a water bath for 45 minutes at 375°F

Remove from water bath as soon as possible and place on a rack to cool
Refrigerate

Serving suggestion:
Top with ½ teaspoon chia seeds
Top with crumbled raw walnuts
Top with crumbled raw pecan pieces

Since I must confess that I'm not into desserts, I thought I would direct you to those who make wonderful *raw, no bake desserts*—something different that you may want to try. Those types of desserts are trending in the raw foods dietary movement.

Raw Blueberry Pie
http://www.damyhealth.com/2012/04/raw-blueberry-pie-single-serving-whole

Raw Pecan Pie
http://www.damyhealth.com/2012/09/raw-pecan-pie-vegan-gf/

Vegan Pumpkin Pie Cheesecake
http://www.damyhealth.com/2012/02/vegan-pumpkin-pie-cheesecake/

Vegan Lemon Cheesecake
http://www.onegreenplanet.org/vegan-recipe/lemon-cheesecake/

Numerous No-Bake Cookie Recipes
http://www.damyhealth.com/2011/12/clean-eating-no-bake-cookies/

One of the issues I have with raw, no-bake desserts is that they use coconut oil, which I like to stay away from since I feel it's highly processed oil[258].

Even though I don't bake, I do have some baking tips, especially about binders.

Two seeds, flax and chia, have mucilaginous properties that help in binding ingredients in cookies, quick breads, and some other baked goods. However, flaxseeds need to be ground, and you can grind them in a coffee grinder. The oils in flaxseeds are easily damaged nutritionally, so it's best to grind them before use and keep them refrigerated or in the freezer.

Now here's the baking trick and conversion for substituting ground flaxseeds for eggs: You can substitute 1 Tablespoon of ground flaxseed mixed with 3 Tablespoons of water for 1 egg. However, you cannot use the mixture until it jells, so if you want to try flaxseeds instead of eggs in your baking, prep the flaxseeds before you start your recipe so that the seeds will have jelled by the time you have to add them to the recipe. Flaxseeds don't work in cakes or any recipe that makes a raised product, e.g., cakes, as it does not leaven or raise the batter while in the oven. Use flaxseeds only in banana bread, cookies, and most muffins.

However, there is an informative website for various substitutes that may be of help: http://fatfreevegan.com/substitutes-and-techniques-for-fat-free-cooking/ not only for baking substitutes, but alternatives to use in personal recipes that you may want to convert into healthier ingredients.

The last dessert or baking tip is about whipped cream. You can use heavy, full-fat, *not lite*, canned coconut milk to make whipped coconut

---

258 http://www.tropicaltraditions.com/what_is_virgin_coconut_oil.htm accessed 3-10-15

cream instead of dairy whipped cream. Here's an online tutorial on how to do it.

http://ohsheglows.com/2012/08/30/coconut-whipped-cream-a-step-by-step-photo-tutorial/

Catherine's After Thoughts

Shortly after finishing this book, I experienced a dramatic awakening, plus a reality check, when I heard a radio announcement about how much is being paid for prescription drugs, since I don't use them. It boggled my mind to hear just how sick people apparently are, but also how easily they could avoid most sicknesses, if only they would pay attention to what they stuff into their mouths.

None other than the World Health Organization has stated that diseases related to obesity, diabetes, cardiovascular disease, several forms of cancer, osteoporosis, and dental disease can be attributed to improper nutrition. Remarkably, in its joint report with the FAO on *Diet, Nutrition and the Prevention of Chronic Disease,* we find this:

> *Not all fats are the same, it pays to know the difference. The scientific complexities of these issues should not obscure the simple messages required to orient and guide consumers. People should eat less high-calorie foods, especially foods high in saturated or trans fats and sugar, be physically active, prefer unsaturated fat and use less salt; enjoy fruits, vegetables and legumes; and select foods of plant and marine*

origin. This consumption pattern is not only healthier but more favourable to the environment and sustainable development.[259]

That's what I've been preaching since the early 1980s!

In view of the above WHO statement, I wonder why U.S. citizens, in particular, don't seem to get the message. The radio talking head's comment I heard seemingly was "off the wall" regarding the costs involved in purchasing and consuming inordinate amounts of prescription drugs. Furthermore, I am concerned that no one seems to know—*or probably doesn't want to know*—if there are negative cumulative and/or iatrogenic health problems, plus associated costs, from taking as many as ten prescription drugs.

I had to check out some things to make certain the radio voice didn't get his facts wrong.

Here's an example from just one healthcare insurer, the U.S. government's Centers for Medicare and Medicaid Services (CMS). It estimated that it would pay $263.2 *Billion* in 2012 for retail prescription drugs. CMS is only one insurer, which doesn't include all the other health insurance plans in the USA or the world! So, what were the top ten prescription drugs CMS paid for in 2013?

>   Nexium, a proton pump inhibitor reducing stomach acid
>   Advair Diskus, an inhaler for asthma or COPD
>   Crestor, a statin, cholesterol-lowering drug
>   Abilify, an antidepressant
>   Cymbalta, an SSNRI to treat major depression in adults
>   Spiriva treats asthma and COPD
>   Namenda treats Alzheimer's disease
>   Januvia lowers blood sugar in type 2 diabetes

---

[259] http://www.who.int/dietphysicalactivity/publications/trs916/summary/en/ accessed 4-15-16

Lantus Solostar, an insulin gargline injection
Revlimid, a specific cancer drug

Unbelievable as it may become, healthcare costs just may break the U.S. economy if—or better still—when we can't get a handle on costs as people become overwhelmingly chronically ill.

> *"Major drug companies took hefty price increases in the U.S., in some cases more than doubling listed charges, for widely used medications over the past five years, a Reuters analysis of proprietary data found. Prices for four of the nation's top 10 drugs increased more than 100 percent since 2011, Reuters found. Six others went up more than 50 percent. Together, the price increases on drugs for arthritis, high cholesterol, asthma and other common problems added billions in costs for consumers, employers and government health programs."*
>
> REUTERS, 4/4/2016[260]

With revenue streams like the above, pharmaceutical makers undoubtedly must be welcoming their good fortune at the cost of sick individuals—how unfortunate, in my opinion.

So, what are average prescription costs for an individual like, I wondered. Based upon Express Scripts' data, the average annual prescription costs for 2013 – 2014 were $1,370.00, representing almost 14 percent of an individual's prescription drug costs. Does that mean that the overall average annual prescription cost for an individual in 2013 – 2014 was about $9,786.00? *Caching* go Big Pharma's cash registers.

---

[260] http://www.fool.com/investing/general/2015/12/12/the-average-american-spends-this-much-on-prescript.aspx accessed 4-15-16

But here's where it really becomes frightening, I think. According to Express Scripts, the highest spending members are baby boomers, with a third of its members being treated for at least 10 conditions! Data say 60 percent were taking a minimum of ten different prescription drugs! Some pills costing as high as $1,125.00 per pill.[261]

Did you know that the demand for prescription drugs is highest in the USA—more than anywhere else in the world? I wonder why! Could it be because we are subjected to so many more chemicals in our food and water than most other countries? Take a look at an example of food ingredient labels for the same product, *McDonalds Strawberry Sauce*, ingredients: one sold in the USA; the other, in the United Kingdom.

The USA label states: Strawberries, Sugar, Water, High Fructose Corn Syrup, Natural Strawberry Flavor With Other Natural Flavors (Fruit Source), Citric Acid, Pectin, Sodium Benzoate (Preservative), Carob Bean Gum, Red 40, Calcium Chloride.

The UK label reads: Strawberries (37%), Sugar, Glucose Syrup, Water, Gelling Agent (Pectin), Acidulant (Citric Acid).[262] Quite a difference, I'd say; wouldn't you?

Furthermore, as many chemicals are banned in other countries, they literally are devoured nonchalant-like in the USA. U.S.-produced meats are banned in over 160 countries, yet Americans love them and pig out on processed meats like hot dogs, hamburgers, sausages, and delicatessen.

Another example is formaldehyde-releasing ingredients in cosmetics. However, the classic U.S. health *faux pas* is the FDA's most unfortunate

---

261 Ibid.
262 http://www.100daysofrealfood.com/2013/02/11/food-companies-exploit-americans-with-ingredients-banned-in-other-countries/ accessed 4-15-16

mandate that genetically modified 'phood' must not be labeled in the USA, which apparently resulted from consensus-corporate-science. Apparently, long-term (2 year) rat-feeding tests were not required by FDA, but only 90-day animal test results were presented—and obviously considered dogmatically-scientifically sufficient—for the FDA's approval! I think I'd call that "tobacco science."

In dramatic contrast, the European Union functions by taking into consideration what's called the "Precautionary Principle," whereas it's quite apparent the U.S. federal alphabet agencies really don't give a hoot about the Precautionary Principle, but genuinely kowtow to corporate interests and lobbyists, many of whom write legislation/bills for members of Congress to introduce and pass in order to protect and apparently promote pharmaceutical, chemical, and corporate interests.

The only way out from under heavy prescription drug costs and poor health is "eat to beat disease."

About the Author

As a result of her lifelong interest in Nature and the natural way, Catherine J Frompovich matriculated in *holistic* modalities and *natural* nutrition. During her studies that led to advanced degrees in *Nutrition and Holistic Health Sciences* along with *Certification in Orthomolecular Theory and Practice*, she came to realize how important it is to follow the "owner's manual" that comes with the human body - Nature's intended way of life, living, and healthcare. She spent numerous years in practice as a consulting nutritionist.

Catherine has been a consumer health researcher and advocate since the late 1970s. Now retired, she was in the vanguard of the health and wellness movement based on *holistic health* principles; *natural*, nutritious foods and diet; *complementary and alternative medicine* (CAM); and the wisdom of health and healing as passed down through the years from various cultures.

Nothing, in her opinion, is more valid and categorically proven than healing systems which have withstood the test of time to provide the wisdom of the ages handed down through generations. Now, mainstream science and medicine are beginning to agree with some of Catherine's convictions.

For many years, Catherine was a practicing *natural* nutritionist working with nutrition-minded physicians and their patients to help them realize the importance of a whole foods and plant-based diet, plus lifestyle changes—long before the rather recent trend. That, back then, garnered the pejorative of "Quack," a compliment of sorts, Catherine quips. Nutrition research, journals, science, and even allopathic medicine, rather reluctantly, have embraced what Catherine preached and practiced years before they came on board. "What took them so long," is her question, and "Why?"

Catherine is the author of numerous books dealing with health, wellness, and *natural* nutrition since the 1970s. Currently, several of her books are available on Amazon.com. They include: *Our Chemical Lives And The Hijacking of Our DNA, A Probe Into What's Probably Making Us Sick* (2009); *A Cancer Answer, Holistic BREAST Cancer Management, A Guide to Effective & Non-Toxic Treatments* (2012); *Vaccination Voodoo, What YOU Don't Know About Vaccines* (2013).

Over the years, Catherine's articles have appeared in various journals, publications, magazines, newspapers, Internet sites, and blogs.

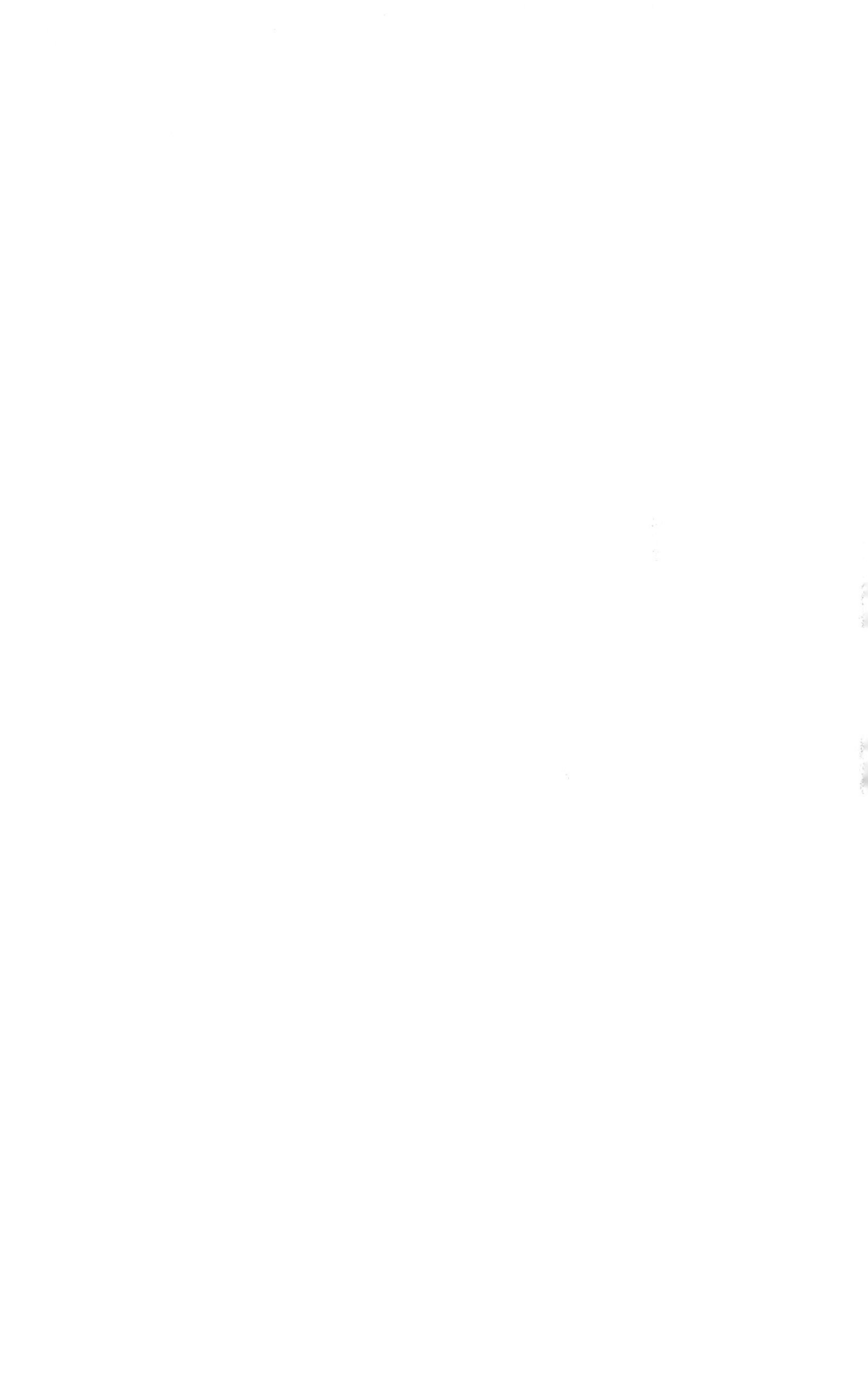

Printed in Great Britain
by Amazon